Weight Loss Surgery

Understanding & Overcoming Morbid Obesity

Life Before, During & After Surgery

Michelle Boasten
FBE Service Network & Network Publishing
Akron, Ohio

Thank You

Jesus	I thank you Lord for blessing me with the opportunity to minister through this book to hurting people.
Frances Roscoe	I thank you Mom for being a friend and supporter. I will always love you.
Adrienne White	I thank you for taking the time to edit this book. Your friendship and love mean so very much to me.
Linda Radak	I thank you Linda for editing this book. I have faith in knowing that your surgery is coming soon. Where there's a will, there's a way!
Chris Markum	I thank you Chris for your contribution. You helped to change my Mom from a critic to a supporter. Your WLS story is one of my favorites! I can't wait to see you flying the friendly skies!
Jamie Anda	What can I say? Every time I look at your before & after pictures I am amazed. You are a beautiful person inside and outside. Thank you for your contribution to this book and for encouraging me in my own WLS journey.
Rick & Janet Armour	I thank you Janet & Rick for all of your encouragement. Your willingness to share has helped and encouraged me and I know it will continue to encourage many more.
Vicki Steinhardt	I thank you Vicki for editing this book. May your husband always know that your attention to detail is a gift from God.
Karen Judd	I thank you "Littermate" Karen for editing this book. I appreciate all of your support and encouragement.
Cecelia Sveda	I am grateful for your help. I could not have submitted this book to the printer without you. Looking for the best graphic designer on the planet? I highly recommend Minx Design at 1-888-GET-MINX (438-6469).
Sherri Booth	I am grateful for your last minute edits at Panera's. Thank you for taking the time to review the book.
Special Thanks	A special word of thanks goes to everyone who shared a quote, edited and reviewed this book. I appreciate your willingness and openness to contribute to this project.
	A special word of thanks goes to everyone who purchased the first printing of this book. Because of your support, this book is a top seller for Barnes & Noble and an Amazon.com top 100 bestseller and #10 in Ohio!

Dedication

This book is dedicated to every person who has ever struggled with morbid obesity. I want you to know that I have walked in your shoes. I understand, first hand, the pain of being misunderstood, prejudged and defined by a morbidly obese frame.

I pray that the words contained in this book will minister to your hurt and begin the healing journey. I want you to find hope to overcome the overwhelming burdens associated with carrying an extra hundred pounds or more.

This project is a sincere labor of love. I thank the hundreds of people who have gone before me on their weight loss surgery journey and had the courage to share their stories. You gave me the courage to share my own story.

Desktop Design & Production: FBE Service Network
Cover Design: Michelle Boasten
Cover Art: © Daryl Benson / Masterfile

Weight Loss Surgery
Understanding & Overcoming Morbid Obesity
Life Before, During & After Surgery

Information for Classification or Cataloging

Boasten, Michelle F.

Weight Loss Surgery: Understanding & Overcoming Morbid Obesity—Life Before, During & After Surgery (2nd Edition)

Weight Loss Surgery; Bariatric Surgery; Obesity Surgery; Weight Loss; Morbid Obesity; Obesity & Overweight; Diet & Nutrition

ISBN: 1-931033-01-3

Disclaimer: This publication is sold with the understanding that the publisher is not engaged in rendering psychological, medical or other professional services. The book is sold without warranties of any kind, express or implied. The publisher and the author disclaim any liability, loss or damage caused by the contents of this book. This book was written for informational purposes, and should not be used as a substitute for consultation with your medical doctor, surgeon or other health care professional. The content in this book is based upon the author's experiences, thoughts and research. Nothing is implied that dictates the outcome of your own experience. You are being provided with the information so that you will be able to make a choice at your own risk. It is your choice whether to act upon any information you have gathered. You should consider this book, the author or its contents educational material and not to be the practice of medicine or to replace consultation with a physician, surgeon, other medical practitioner or health care professional.

To contact the publisher, write to:
FBE Service Network 631 West Exchange Street, Akron, Ohio 44302-1326.

Printed in the USA

Contents

Introduction

*My obesity
story is
not that
different
from
yours…*

My obesity started at age seven. It was the mid 70's and genetic research wasn't what it is today. I was born to "normal size" parents who believed what many people today believe despite the genetic findings. My parents believed that I was getting fat because I ate too much. Of course, at age seven, my parents controlled what I ate. They did the shopping, the cooking and the serving. In addition, they controlled all the money. If they didn't give me money, I didn't have any. They assumed that I must have been eating somewhere. The ridicule started early in my life and with it came all of the feelings of shame, guilt, rejection and embarrassment. All of these negative emotions and more were heaped on my seven year old soul.

I watched my father blame my mother for my obesity and my mother blamed me. The blaming hurt. And even though I am a grown woman, I still feel a small sting of pain when I think about those memories.

By age 11, I was taken to the pediatrician and put on Ionamin, better known as my first amphetamine. I lost weight, but this would turn out to be the first roller coaster, yo-yo diet pattern that would characterize my life for the next twenty-some years.

Like most morbidly obese people, I blamed myself repeatedly for gaining the weight back. I'd beat myself up emotionally. But in my heart of hearts, I knew that I didn't eat "that much more" than my "thin or normal sized" friends. I even made the mistake of sharing that with my mother. She (at the time) couldn't, wouldn't or didn't go along with my theory.

I heard about weight loss surgery in the 1980's and the term being thrown around was "stomach stapling." I must say that the term "stomach stapling" sounded about as appealing as jaw wiring. I never considered either approach for weight loss for me. Even though I knew I didn't eat that differently from my normal sized peers, I held on to that dreaded societal and familial philosophy about obesity that was engraved on my psyche at age seven. That philosophy told me that my obesity was my fault. My thought about stomach stapling and jaw wiring was that if I had to resort to such drastic measures, then I really was out of control. Which would give more credence to the belief system that says fat people are obviously already out of control. Fortunately, I didn't choose jaw wiring or stomach stapling because, like all other "diets" and "gimmicks," the weight comes back on with avengeance!

I remember watching one of the national evening news shows and one of the segments was about leptin. There was some amazing breakthrough that showed that the amount and presence of this body chemical or protein contributed to obesity. Later in the report, they showed the standard lab rat and then one that was injected with more leptin. That second rat was morbidly obese. I sat up and paid attention to that report because it was the first time science had backed up my own personal theory that my obesity was not my fault.

I started to closely follow the obesity science and research studies in the mid 1990's. During this same time period, a dear friend of mine, who was also morbidly obese, shared that she met a couple of women who had gastric bypass surgery. She told me that they had lost weight and they were able to keep it off. The whole sound of it harkened back to my thoughts of "stomach stapling" and I actually discouraged her from the idea of having surgery, mostly because of what I learned in nursing school about gastric bypass surgery. I remember learning about the gastric bypass complications of decades past when gastric bypass patients were well known for long ICU stays and even death.

It wasn't until the 1999 Internet hosted surgery of Carnie Wilson that I recognized that weight loss surgery was for me. By this time, I was so convinced that my obesity was genetic that I had developed my own theories about my obesity. And since nobody really knows what causes morbid obesity, my theory was just as good as anyone else. I thank God I arrived at the decision that weight loss surgery (WLS) was for me.

I found all sorts of good information on the Internet, but I couldn't find a single guide to walk me through my WLS Journey. That is why you are reading this book, because I couldn't find the very book that you are holding in your hands right now.

My WLS Journey has been and continues to be a wonderful experience. Surgery is serious, but I liken the experience and the excitement of this particular surgery to someone getting corrective or life saving surgery. I was looking forward to being anatomically corrected.

What WLS did for me is give me hope. Hope is the whole-hearted belief that something GREAT is going to happen. It is the joyful anticipation of a fulfilled end in your favor. Hope is a close cousin to faith. I think that the best thing that this experience has done for me is given me hope to overcome the trappings of obesity.

> *Hope is the whole-hearted belief that something GREAT is going to happen. It is the joyful anticipation of a fulfilled end in your favor.*

This surgery took me off that dreaded roller coaster and validated what I knew at age seven! Morbid obesity is not my fault. I suspect for many of you reading, your morbid obesity is not your fault either. Nobody can make you believe that, you have to come to that conclusion for yourself.

It feels fantastic to no longer beat myself up. Eight weeks after surgery, even though I was still morbidly obese, I felt good enough to exercise. And I'm actually starting to like it! That is a miracle! For the first time in my life, I am going to have the lifelong benefits of living in a normal size body and I am free from the fear that the weight will return.

For those of you who will disagree with my thoughts, beliefs, theories and philosophies, that's fine with me. I don't expect the world to agree with me nor is it a goal of mine. I simply want to encourage those who were or are in the same boat that I was in. I firmly believe that some part of this book will touch you.

I pray that this book is exactly what you need in your WLS Journey. Consider this a divine appointment.

Sincerely,
Michelle

Chapter One

Chris' story is great. She was featured in the January 8, 2001 edition of First Magazine. Her story is a dream come true. Chris worked for an airline as a telephone reservation agent. As she'd answer the calls one by one, she realized that this job was the only job she could get with the airline weighing in at nearly 300 pounds. She learned about weight loss surgery and her life transformation after surgery allowed her to fulfill a dream. After losing 100 pounds, she was approached by the airline to attend flight attendant school. Today, Chris is a full-time flight attendant with aspirations to attend flight school soon.

"The best thing WLS has done for me is given me my life back. It's given me the opportunity to do the things I never thought I could do. I can't even begin to explain what this has done for me overall. It's truly amazing and I thank God everyday for the changes that have happened in my life in the last two years. I never would have thought it was possible."

Chris Markum
Flight Attendant
Laparoscopic MGB, 3/25/1999

Did You Choose Obesity Or Did Obesity Choose You

Determining Your Own Obesity Philosophy

Determining your destiny about your morbid obesity has to first begin by shaping your own philosophy about obesity. What you believe about your morbid obesity will impact how you respond to it. Developing your destiny about obesity means taking control of your own obesity philosophy.

This book was written for people who are morbidly obese. How do you know if you are morbidly obese? Well there are charts and formulas that I could share, but I don't want to use them yet. I want you to ask yourself this basic question. Are you living in a "normal size body?" Does the size of your body create mental and physical burdens that most normal size people have no clue exist? Things like not fitting in chairs or the inability to shop in a "normal size" store. If you are not morbidly obese, weight loss surgery is probably not for you. I won't discourage you from reading further; I think it will be insightful. But if you are a morbidly obese person, this book is beyond insightful, it's validating.

We know that gluttony and overeating will lead to weight gain and in some cases it will lead to obesity, but we all know someone who can eat and won't gain - - we hate them. Or at least I do, or did. I can admit that I have been envious of their God-given "Road Runner" metabolism and down right angry that mine moved more like a garden slug. It took some maturing, and now I realize that everybody has God-given gifts, skills, talents and abilities. You may have gotten stuck with a slow metabolism (and surgery won't change that), but you have some other gifts.

It is terribly important that you start your journey with a good look at what you believe about your obesity. This theory or philosophy, whether you recognize it or not, will drive your decisions, actions and reactions about your weight. I am going to give you some difficult questions to ask yourself. You will address areas that you should carefully give some thought. In Chapter Two, I'll share my personal theory about morbid obesity.

It's really important to understand that nobody, but our Creator knows what's really going on inside our bodies. Medical science has not uncovered the many mysteries that our bodies hold, and I suspect that if I live a hundred more lifetimes, the mysteries will still not be unraveled.

With that, I want you to take a journey back in time; it may even be in your childhood. I would like to start with this question. When did you first learn about fat and skinny? The problem is, most people cannot answer that. Knowledge of body size or any other physical characteristic, like hair color, skin color or eye color are all visually observed and I suppose these things are recognized when we were able to see, even though they may not mean anything to us. We can tell from infants that they recognize their mothers by sight. Even a toddler can point at a picture of their mom and say "Mommy". Mommy may have been fat, skinny or somewhere in between, and the toddler may not have realized it, but Mommy's body size is just one of the physical cues to let the toddler know that this is Mommy.

Since it is hard to tell when you first learned about fat and skinny, it may be easier to ask another question. When you were a child what did you think about obesity? If that's too hard, what did you think about obesity in junior high or high school? Somewhere between toddler age and school age, it is evident that strong, often very negative messages about obesity are sent our way and this is when we start to shape our philosophy and theory about obesity. I suspect that many people hold on to that same philosophy about obesity for the rest of their lives. It wouldn't be so bad if the philosophy weren't so damaging (we'll talk about that later).

Whether you were the "fat kid" or not, there's a good chance that you remember the "fat kid." You may not remember the fat kid's name, but if you weren't the fat kid, I bet you didn't want to be subject to the teasing and ridicule of the "fat kid." Maybe you did the teasing, maybe not. Either way, the teasing about body size is directly related to the messages ingrained about obesity. Somewhere, somehow, some way, the child doing the teasing has learned, fat equals something funny. I strongly suspect that this is probably where the fat and jolly myth got started. But the truth is that, someone's fat made the others jolly. But the fat person, especially a child, is rarely jolly when made the object of such ridicule.

I'm not a psychologist or a psychiatrist, and I don't know how much damage is done to a child when so much ridicule is hurled at them, but I do know that each person has a measure of mental health, and when that threshold is exceeded, something has to give way. I also know, from my own "fat kid" experience, that there are some skills that are developed as a result of this ridicule. While I was being teased and tormented, I didn't know that anything good could come out of that, but now that I am an adult, I know that suffering really does bring about proven character.

Lessons from the fat kid...

The "fat kids" learn many valuable lessons early in life. The experience of being teased and left out are hard, but what's learned is invaluable and irreplaceable. As you read them, you may at first think, these are horrible lessons, but you will find that they are lessons we all must learn, it's just a matter of what life chooses to use to get the message across to you.

Emotional Control
I knew that I couldn't cry in front of all those kids, or my suffering would have been magnified. In fact, I thought at times it was the goal of my tormentors to see me "crack". Have you ever felt this way on a job? Crying is healthy, but there's a place to show emotion and a place not to show emotion. I'll bet Bill Clinton cried many times when he was going through that impeachment process, but every time that man got on television his eyes were dry. Learning when and where to show emotion and learning to exercise some emotional control is a skill that's needed every single day. How many times have you been angry with someone and you knew you should clam up instead of blow up? When people don't know how to deal with their emotions, they are unstable. I credit my fat kid experience for teaching me to exercise some emotional control.

Stand For What Is Right
Early on, I learned that there were kids who would tease me and there were kids who would be silent, but then there was that third group. Those were the kids who knew that teasing was wrong, and when I couldn't speak up, they spoke for me. I appreciated those kids and it taught me something about friendship. They also taught me how to defend what was right and to do it without shame knowing that backlash might be coming my way just because of the position I took. It taught me that being right or correct may not always be the easy choice, in fact it could be down

right difficult, but standing on principle was the right thing to do. I credit having some backbone to my "fat kid" years.

How To Decipher Character
Most kids know that teasing and name-calling are wrong. Most mothers teach "If you can't say something good, don't say anything at all". When I was teased, it was easy to tell whom not to trust, it was my tormentors. Early on, I learned that those who stood by in silence, but still befriended my tormentors were taking a stand. It was taking a position of approval; it was just a quiet stand. I learned that people could give hearty approval through silence. I also learned that this group was not trustworthy. This is an excellent lesson. Birds of a feather flock together. You can tell the character of a person by the company they keep.

How To Forgive
While at times I did loathe some of the teasing kids, I did learn to forgive. I learned that some people really are ashamed for what they have done and they want to make amends. I am glad that I didn't hold grudges and God knows this is a skill that's needed for any human relationship. Whether intentional or not, somebody is going to hurt you. Holding the anger inside and being unwilling to forgive will eat you alive. Early on in life I had to practice forgiveness and I owe my first forgiveness experiences to the "fat kid years".

From youth, we learn that fatness or obesity is associated with being unattractive, lazy, ugly, dirty stupid and lacking control. I remember watching a news report where young children were being polled. Second and third graders were asked to choose whether they would want to be fat or blind. And most of them said they would rather be blind instead of being fat. This means that whatever messages are being sent, learned and digested by society permeate the children at a very young age. Especially if they'd choose to be blind over being fat!

Can you list some examples of cartoons or other forms of media that depict fatness or obesity with a negative stereotype? Do you agree with this stereotype? Are you unattractive or lazy? Do you lack control? Are you ugly, dirty or stupid? Even if you do see yourself this way, do you know a fat or obese person who is attractive? What about someone fat who exhibits a position of power that requires lots of control? Do you know any smart fat people? If you don't, allow me to introduce myself. I am fat and I am also pretty and smart. I am definitely not lazy, I work all the time! I can admit though that I didn't like being a large person. I didn't like the physical and mental burdens associated with being morbidly obese.

I'd like to turn your thoughts to your own morbidly obese experience. Go through the list of mental and physical burdens associated with being morbidly obese and highlight what applies to you.

The Mental Challenges

- I lack self-confidence
- I don't feel good about the way I look
- I want to be free from obvious public ridicule about my size
- I often feel embarrassed about my size
- I want to be free from worrying about obesity related health problems
- I have obesity related fears about being accepted
- I get tired of hearing "You have such a pretty face"
- I have lied about something related to my weight
- I have turned down an invitation because of my weight
- I have felt shame about my weight
- I have felt guilt about my weight
- I have been rejected because of my weight
- I am very self-conscious about my weight
- I know people treat me differently because of my size
- I am tired of being pre-judged based on my weight
- I fear that I will not live to see my children grow up
- I am embarrassed that my children will be teased about having a fat parent
- I am ashamed to look at myself naked or have others see me undressed
- I won't see a doctor because I am too large
- Summer clothing is embarrassing to wear, especially shorts and swimsuits
- I try to cover up my body so that no one will see the skin on my arms and legs
- I am unable to look at a full-length reflection of my body
- I quickly get away from full-length mirrors where others can see my reflection
- I run from the camera
- When I must be in a photo I try to hide in the back row

The Physical Challenges

- I have physical limitations because of my weight
- I can't enjoy sex fully at the size I am
- I want to wear normal size clothes and shop in a normal size store
- I lack energy
- I have experienced shortness of breath without a lot of exertion
- I wake up in the middle of the night gasping for air due to sleep apnea
- I am unable to run, jump and play with my children
- I sweat more than I should
- I have body aches, especially in the joints
- Movement is hard for me
- I can't bend over
- I can't stoop down and get back up
- If I sit on the floor, getting up is difficult or even impossible
- Pantyhose are hard to wear and get on
- I cannot cross my legs above the ankles
- I have had trouble fitting in restaurant booths
- I have had trouble fitting in seats with arms, including theater seats, airline seats, the dentists' chair, amusement park rides, school desks, sporting events, barber chairs and more
- I have ankles that are not normal looking
- I have to use seat belt extensions or go without using a seat belt putting myself at risk
- I have sat in a chair that was unable to hold my weight
- I have opted to stand instead of sitting in a chair because I thought it would not hold my weight
- I am unable to play sports due to my size, lack of energy or embarrassment about how I would look or be teased
- I have been limited by weight restrictions including horseback riding, ladders, exercise equipment and more
- I have checked the weight limit sign on the elevator
- I have weighed more than a scale will measure
- I have developed skin rashes associated with my obesity
- I have problems with a very large abdomen; like spilling things, getting wet, driving or bending
- I have had to use the handicapped stall in a public restroom
- I have been unable to use a turnstile properly or at all
- I have had trouble fitting in aisles, including turning sideways to fit through
- I do not have a neck or jaw line
- I have had trouble fitting into hospital gowns, hairdresser smocks or the dreaded gynecologist paper robes

- I am unable to tie my shoes
- I am unable to wear normal jewelry like necklaces, bracelets, anklets and watches
- I want to wear clothes without elastic or stretch quality
- I can't wear boots
- I can't wear pull up socks
- I can't fit into the back seat of a two-door car or I have trouble getting out of them
- I do not have a lap; my large thighs are like a sliding slope
- I have trouble with urinary incontinence
- I have trouble with toileting hygiene from not being able to reach
- I am unable to fit in a standard bathtub or a shower stall

It is not easy living with these mental and physical burdens. Life presents plenty of challenges and when you add these to the list it just makes life harder. Or at least it did for me. If you are like most obese people, you have done more than fantasized about living life in a normal size body; you have tried a number of ways to get into a normal size body. Below are a list of diets and gimmicks to "help" obese people lose weight and live life in a normal size body. Highlight the ones that you've tried. If you have been able to maintain weight loss using one of these "diets or gimmicks", contact the National Institute of Health. They did a 17-year study and it concluded that less than 1% of morbidly obese people were able to lose weight and keep it off. If your diet isn't listed, add it to the list.

The Diets & Gimmicks

- Fasting; Starvation
- Acupuncture
- Hypnosis
- Low Carb, High Protein Diet: Atkins, Sugar Busters, The Zone, Carbohydrate Addicts
- Low Fat High Carb Diet
- Low Fat, No Fat Diet
- American Diabetic Association Diet
- Beverly Hills Diet
- Fit For Life
- Self-Induced Vomiting; Bulimia
- The Cabbage Soup Diet
- Weight Loss Camps; Spas; Structure House
- The Diet Centers; Physician's Weight Loss; Jenny Craig; Weight Watchers; TOPS; Weigh Down Workshop; Formu-3; NutriSystem
- The Grapefruit Diet
- The Vinegar Diet

- The Lemon Juice Diet
- Work Out Videos; Tae Bo; Jane Fonda; Richard Simmons; Kathy Smith; Susan Powter
- Richard Simmons Deal-A-Meal or Food Card Diets
- Hospital Diets; Mayo Clinic; Cleveland Clinic; Duke Diet
- The Rice Diet
- Shakes, Mixes and Drinks: Medifast; Optifast; SlimFast
- Metabolife; Metabolite
- Calorad
- BioSlim
- Prescription Amphetamines; Phen-Fen; Redux; Meridia; Xenical; Diuretics
- Private Cooks, Counselors, Trainers
- Overeaters Anonymous
- The Pritikin Diet
- Tony Robbins Motivational Tapes; Any motivational tapes
- The Scarsdale Diet
- Over The Counter Diet Pills; Dexatrim; Water Pills; Laxatives; Appetite Suppressant Gum and Candy
- Herbal remedies
- Jaw Wiring
- Stomach Stapling (no bypass)
- Plastic Sweat Suits
- Your own made up low calorie diet
- Your own form of exercise

This list can continue on and on. I just listed the most popular and well-known methods of trying to lose weight. The reason I list these diets are to show you that at some point, you wanted the weight off. I also use this list to show you that each diet can represent failure and like the other mental stresses in your life, repeated failures are not healthy. The emotions that come from morbid obesity are hard to deal with. Next, spend some time going through this list of emotions and see if you can recall a time when you felt the emotion as it relates to your body size.

Have you felt...

- Guilt
- Shame
- Embarrassment
- Disappointment
- Despair
- Rejection
- Pain

- Ridicule
- Humiliation
- Mortified
- Isolated
- Ignored
- Hopeless
- Heartbroken
- Fear
- Panic
- Discarded
- Betrayed
- Like You Were a Failure

All of these feelings are hard to experience. Life in a morbidly obese body seems to invite these feelings. While the lists may bring back a flood of painful memories, it is important to take this inventory to take a hard look at what life is like in a morbidly obese body.

Earlier in this chapter, I pointed out that the societal beliefs about obesity are damaging. In the Introduction of this book, I describe how pervasive is the thought that obesity is a matter of gluttony and eating despite the current research findings about the genetic links associated with morbid obesity. What makes this thought pattern so damaging, is that many people buy into it and it feeds into deeper feelings of guilt and shame instead of pointing to the only known solution that will end your cycle of morbid obesity and allow you to maintain lifelong weight loss and live in a normal size body. Sure you may have ate the "wrong things", but so do many normal size people. Sure you may not exercise, and when I was 372 pounds I couldn't Tae, let alone Bo! But I didn't eat my way to 372 pounds! I didn't ride the Twinkie Express to Morbidly Obese Land. I didn't choose obesity... it chose me.

Chapter Two

"For as long as I can remember I have always wanted to fit in and have friends. I wanted to be a "normal" teenager. But I wasn't. I was overweight and that effected everything I did or didn't do. I didn't wear shorts outside my house because I hated my legs. I wouldn't go to any school dances or parties, I wasn't invited anywhere, and basically had very few friends who cared about what happened to me and how my life was going."

"During this whole time I was desperately searching for a way out of this body, this prison. I hate to admit it, but from ages 14 to 17 I was really depressed and had thoughts of killing myself, but luckily I wised up and just knew that God would help me if I truly wanted it. And I didn't expect Him to do all the work. October, 1998 was when I first heard and read about weight loss surgery and at first it scared me a lot. But after I did months of research and praying I knew I had to trust God and take this leap. Basically the benefits of this surgery outweigh all the risks."

Jamie Anda
http://freewill.tzo.com/~jamie
Open RNY, 1/5/2000

God Works In Mysterious Ways...

*My
Own
Medical
Theory*

After all of the research, reports, studies and findings, I have been left with the fact that the researchers agree on one thing. That thing is that overeating or gluttony alone does not cause morbid obesity. There's a genetic component and behavior component.

The truth about obesity, morbid obesity anyway, is that no one has unraveled the full mystery yet. Genetic research is slowly unveiling what has been hidden from humans. I suspect that if I lived another hundred lifetimes, I don't think we will ever know what really causes some people's body to grow and store so much more fat than others.

When I let go of that damaging societal view of obesity, it freed me to embrace my own philosophy and theory. I stopped beating up myself, and I vowed that I would no longer be the victim of counterfeit diets and gimmicks.

I've tried all sorts of experiments on my own body including fasting, starvation, eating only protein, abstaining from "fat", eating only at certain times of the day, eating specially prepared meals and more. I was obsessed with the scale. I would weigh myself several times a day. Over and over and over again I did this. I even followed the American Diabetic Association's (ADA) 800-calorie per day diet and I found myself "maintaining", but not losing.

I am a Christian. I really thought there were some "spiritual" things going on. Was it some kind of "demonic" thing going on in my body or what? Did I not trust in God enough? Was my faith not working? What was it? My prayer style is very "conversational," it's more than a monologue. I would ask God to please tell me why my body is this size. I know I'm not eating so much more than others that I should be this large. What gives? What's wrong with me? Over and over I'd ask the Lord to reveal something to me.

There was a time when the psychological community introduced childhood abuse as a reason for obesity. They said if you've been sexually, mentally, physically or emotionally abused, food was the way you were dealing with the pain and that is why some people are fat. Maybe this is true, but I wasn't the victim of child abuse. Once I was at an Overeaters Anonymous meeting and a size two woman stood up and cried and cried because she ate a piece of chocolate cake. I don't want to make light of her pain, but I knew this was the wrong meeting for me. I wanted to cry because I couldn't fit in the movie theater seat without getting bruises on my thighs and here she was a size two! Something was not right about us both being in that meeting, so I left.

I remember coming to the conclusion that there was something "different" about my body. It seemed to be "obesity-prone," but I didn't know why. Yes I like food, LOVE food, but so do skinny people. Food is a source of socialization, associated with good times, holidays and such, not to mention the taste of some foods is WONDERFUL. Some people prefer food to sex (usually women).

God was the ONLY person I could talk to. I knew all along that I didn't eat continually. I would watch these horrible news stories on CNN or 20/20. The reporter would show a person who was about 800 or 1000+ pounds locked up in their home, a hostage of their own body and they needed a crane or something extraordinary to get them out of the house. They had lost the function of mobility and they were literally too big to do anything physical. With an interview forthcoming, they would report that a relative or close friend would be fixing them meals to the tune of a dozen eggs and a loaf of toast every morning. I can assure you that if I were in this physical condition my relatives and friends, especially my mother, wouldn't feed me birdseed let alone a real meal.

I refused to buy sweets and my friends have to bring their own food when they come to visit me, because I don't have anything to feed them. They will testify to this, so will my mother and father (if he were still living). He used to say, "I don't know where you are hiding the food, cause it sure ain't in the kitchen." That was followed up with this "I don't know how you got this big with no food here at the house." But I wasn't hiding food. I don't want to give the false impression that I didn't eat. I did eat. I just didn't cook. Just like several of my friends and peers, but the result was far different. I ballooned, they maintained. See the difference.

The more I experimented with the diets and the gimmicks the more I became convinced that the diets weren't working for me. Then one day while praying, it became confirmed in my spirit that MY BODY WAS DIFFERENT. I cried and moaned and BEGGED God for a miracle. I wanted Him to change my DNA, right then and there, but He didn't, and that's okay. This gave me something to keep praying about. Like a whining child or a nagging wife I asked over and over and over again. "Change my DNA, restructure it, you created it; you have the power to do it!" But He didn't. Instead, God allowed me to have this very DNA as a vehicle to allow me to show others that obesity is not their fault.

I started to research weight loss surgery on the Internet. The more I studied the genetic findings and the work of the medical research community, it led me to the same conclusion that God had already confirmed in my spirit. I was different and there were real documented scientific findings to back me up! I felt double confirmed. Confirmed by God, then by man.

I am a registered nurse. I had to take a myriad of science courses in college, and I learned about the body's communication system. It is nothing short of

God was the ONLY person I could talk to.

amazing. Did you know that the body communicates with itself continually? Though you may take a nap, the work going on inside the body never really sleeps. Twenty-four seven the brain sends messages out to the cells and the cells send messages back to the brain. Up and down the spinal column through nerves with Morse Code like impulses communication is going on all the time.

Our body is made up of microscopic cells. Our cells work like little tiny bodies inside our body. Like us, our cells get hungry. They communicate to the brain and send hunger messages that say "Hey, we need some food!" The brain then talks to the stomach and it tells it to ache. That's our signal or message to eat. Once the food is consumed, it travels through the digestive system and the food is broken down into its smallest elements so that the cells can eat it.

Before going on, let me give you a small anatomy lesson. I'll give this anatomy lesson later on in greater detail. When you eat, food enters the mouth, goes down the esophagus, into the stomach and out to the small intestine. The small intestine has three parts: the duodenum, the jejunum and the ileum. After food leaves the small intestine, it enters the large intestine, also known as the colon and then we flush it away.

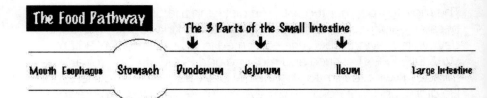

The Food Pathway

The 3 Parts of the Small Intestine

Mouth Esophagus Stomach Duodenum Jejunum Ileum Large Intestine

When the food is in the stomach and passed on to the small intestine, there should be a message from the brain telling the small intestine, particularly the duodenum, how much "nutrition" to keep and how much to let go. So if the cells are full on 5% of the food, the message should be communicated to hold onto 5% and let go of the 95%. Because the body is an efficient machine, a little extra nutrition should be stored "as fat" for a rainy day. This is how the body works for the normal person, but not those of us with "different" genetics.

Those of us with the "special genetics" have some communication problems going on that result in a whole lot of storage. We have enough fat stored for more than a rainy day; our morbid obese body is equipped for a full-fledged hurricane! I don't know where the communication breakdown begins or ends. Remember, it all starts with the communication from the cells when they tell the brain "Hey, I'm hungry". I am going to offer four scenarios that may explain where the communication problem lies. I don't know if any are correct or not. It's my theory and I'm sticking to it!

Scene One, Act One
The Cells Are Lying

Maybe the cells aren't hungry, but they are just plain greedy. The message sent to the brain is that the cells are hungry when they really aren't hungry at all. Likewise, the cells could be lying about how much nutrition they actually need. The cells may only need 5% of the nutrition, but they tell the brain they need 50%.

Scene Two, Act One
The Brain Is Not Telling It Like It Is

It could be that the brain is lying to the duodenum. Maybe the cells are telling the truth and the brain tells the duodenum "The cells need 5% nutrition, but give them 50% nutrition". In this case, the brain is overriding the will of the cells.

Scene Three, Act One
The Intestine is Hard of Hearing or Has a Mind of Its Own

Maybe the cells and brain have communicated correctly, but the duodenum says "I'm going to do my own thing. I don't have to cooperate with you Mr. Brain". And instead of holding on to 5% of the nutrition, it chooses to hold on to 50%.

Scene Four, Act One
The Messengers Are Running Interference and the Brain, Cells and Intestines Are All Telling the Truth

Remember that the messages that are sent and received are sent over nerve channels and pathways. These pathways are the message couriers. Maybe the cells, brain and duodenum are all trying to send a true message, but the couriers are running interference by changing the message and sending something that wasn't intended.

In Conclusion...

I do know this much. If you eat way too much food, like a dozen eggs a day or a loaf of toast, you will gain weight. But for those of you who know you are not packing in a dozen eggs or a loaf of toast, but find yourself grossly obese, please stop beating up on yourself, please stop dieting and get some real help, which is weight loss surgery. It provides a real life solution (until they find a way to alter the genes).

Don't Tell The Paralytic That Walking is Easy...

I have never been paralyzed. From the moment I started walking, at around 8 or 9 months, I've always been able to walk. Walking, like any gross motor skill is controlled by the nervous system. When the brain tells the leg to move, a message is sent down the spinal cord, through the nerves and out to the muscles of the leg. When your nervous system is well functioning, the movement of the leg will be smooth and coordinated. But when the nervous system is not functioning well, the leg will move erratically and spastically with jerky movements. This can make walking difficult if not impossible altogether.

Our nervous system controls more than just our gross motor abilities. It controls everything we do! It even plays a role in our obesity. Thanks to your nervous system, you take walking for granted. Walking is so easy that nearly all one year olds have mastered the ability to walk. But if the nerves that carry the message from the brain to the legs are cut or are severely damaged for whatever reason, walking is not an easy task.

A toddler or a young child doesn't understand the mechanisms of the nervous system. It would be understandable for a toddler to ask a paralytic to walk with them, but the paralytic can't walk. Imagine for a moment that the toddler grows into adulthood and never understands that the reason they are able to walk is because of their well-functioning nervous system. Picture this adult telling the paralytic "All you have to do is get up". I can hear them say the Nike mantra "Just Do It!" It would be nuts for the walking person to tell the paralytic to just get up, walking is easy, it's a matter of will power. Wouldn't it?

Well that's what the diet industry and weight loss gimmick folks are doing to the morbidly obese. Through books, tapes, videos, pills and programs, the "walking" normal size people are telling the "paralytic" morbidly obese to just do it! Their message is that losing weight and keeping it off is easy if you just do 1-2-3. See? It's like telling the paralytic to just put one foot in front of the other and off you go. See how easy it is?

I believe that morbidly obese people have an impaired nervous system, just like the paralytic has an impaired nervous system. Your morbid obesity is not caused by a lack of will power. Genetics, medical problems, environment, psychology and learned behaviors all contribute and play a role in your morbid obesity. You need to stop blaming yourself and stop listening to those "walking" people tell the paralytic that walking is easy. Willpower will not repair an impaired nervous system. The last time history recorded a paralytic walk upon command was when Jesus healed the cripple.

Chapter Three

"I paid fifty bucks to go see the Nutcracker On Ice a couple years ago and I had to sit on the steps because I couldn't fit in the seat. I was so embarrassed I thought I was gonna throw up and I ended up crying through half the show."

Karla Grubb
Open RNY, 1/31/2001

"Could I have lost weight without WLS? Sure, but the chance of keeping it off or maintaining the weight loss was about the same chance that Bill Gates has of qualifying for food stamps..."

Mikayla Francine
www.myminigastricbypass.com
Laparascopic Billroth II, 10/25/2000

Drastic ?

> **dras·tic**
> *adjective*
> Severe or radical in nature; extreme
> Taking effect violently or rapidly
> [Greek drastikos, active,
> from drastos, to be done, from dran, to do.]

In Chapter One, I explained that your philosophy about obesity will drive how you respond to your obesity and even how you respond to the thought of weight loss surgery.

If you agree with society's obesity philosophy that obesity is an issue of gluttony, then it is likely that you may think that weight loss surgery is drastic. In fact, each time I read a news story or report about weight loss surgery, the word drastic is in it. Is there justification for using the adjective drastic? Where does that word come from and why is it linked to weight loss surgery?

If you hold the belief that obesity surgery is purely for cosmetic purposes (which it is not and we'll discuss that later), then obesity surgery should be put in the category of a face-lift or a "nose job." But nobody calls these surgeries drastic do they? Instead, our beauty and youth crazed culture applauds and supports cosmetic surgery.

By contrast, let's say that you believe that obesity surgery is medically necessary (which it is). No other medically necessary surgery is called drastic. My dad had colon polyps removed. Nobody called that drastic. My friend's son had tubes surgically implanted in his ears to drain an infection. Nobody called that drastic. My mother had knee surgery to repair torn cartilage. Nobody called that drastic. Why didn't anybody call these surgeries drastic?

The reason is because surgery is medically indicated and surgery is the appropriate course of treatment.

When is surgery considered drastic?

I am certain that way back when, somebody came up with the idea to cut the body open, repair something inside and close the body back up. Surgery is so commonplace today, that it's obvious that we can't really think it's drastic or it wouldn't be so common. But back when the idea of surgery was first introduced, somebody had to raise some sort of objection. Surely somebody raised the concerns of bleeding to death, unbearable pain and infection. Thank God the surgeons kept forging ahead until the benefits of surgery outweighed the risks. So much so that thousands of people are being operated on every single day.

Why is obesity surgery considered drastic?

I submit to you that the ONLY reason obesity surgery is considered drastic is because society believes that your morbid obesity is caused by your lack of self-control. Somebody is thinking that the only reason you are getting surgery is because you have no self-control. These same people are quick to say "you're taking the easy way out". Well I have just one thing to say to them. If this is the easy way out, the road to get in here was paved with HELL itself. Just go back to Chapter One and see what feelings and experiences one has to deal with to get into this "morbid obesity club". In addition I want to tell these people that if surgery is the "easy way out", I don't want to go out like I came in. I don't want to leave this earth morbidly obese. (Did you know that some people need special caskets because they don't fit in the regular size?) I must tell you that weight loss surgery is no "easy way out" (we'll talk about that later on).

This cynical belief system is no more than a jab to the fat person and a skewer into the philosophy that obesity is not your fault. I have chosen not to fight these cynics. I allow them to say whatever they like. I have learned not to listen. This is a lesson I picked up from my "fat kid years."

What I think is drastic is remaining morbidly obese. Morbid obesity puts you at a much higher risk for type two diabetes, hypertension, depression, some types of cancer, joint dysfunction, arthritis, gout, orthopedic problems and poor self-esteem. And this is not a theory or a philosophy. These findings are well known and well documented facts. I didn't want to be at a two to ten times greater risk of becoming a diabetic or having cardiac problems. But even more, I didn't know how much longer I would be able to endure the physical and mental burdens associated with being morbidly obese. Remember I said that everybody has a breaking point. And nobody really knows what that breaking point looks like.

I don't want to make it seem as though surgery isn't serious. It is SERIOUS, but not drastic. The truth, for me anyway, is that the risks of the surgical complications were much less than the complications associated with remaining morbidly obese.

Is It Normal To Be Afraid?

Anybody undergoing surgery will have some natural fears. They are normal, they are understandable and they are expected. Surgery, for anything, including something as simple as a tooth extraction carry risks. I once learned that any good thing taken to the extreme would no longer be good. Fear is a God-given emotion. Having a healthy amount of fear protects us from danger and harm. I fully respect your fears. But fear taken to the extreme is paralyzing. This is called the "Paralysis of Analysis". You can analyze something so much that you become paralyzed with fear. All surgery, including gastric bypass surgery carries a risk of something going wrong, but often the fears associated with gastric bypass surgery aren't about the surgery itself, but the fear of living in a brand new body. That is a justifiable and understandable fear. For many of us, fat has been with us what seems to be our entire lives. There are obvious unknown elements associated with being a normal size when living large has been the only life you've known. As you come closer to the decision that gastric bypass surgery is for you, your fears will give way to calmness, assurance and peace. When this assurance settles in, you are ready for surgery.

Telling Others

As you arrive at the weight loss surgery decision, you will have to share your decision with someone. This decision is too important to keep it to yourself. As I arrived at the decision that weight loss surgery was for me, I observed how the people in my life responded. I labeled them supporters, critics and cynics. I don't know where you are in your weight loss surgery journey. But talking to others about this surgery is an issue at every stage, especially when the weight starts falling off. Even the casual strangers in your life, like the grocery store clerk will ask,

"How did you lose all that weight?" Again, your philosophy and understanding about obesity will drive how you respond. For now, I want you to make a list of all the people closest to you. Include the people who you interact with on a regular basis. Your list should include people at work or some of your neighbors. Include your doctor on this list as well. Read the descriptions below and next to each name, jot whether they are a supporter, a critic or a cynic.

The Supporters
The supporter wants the best for you. They will be willing to listen. They are teachable and they will be open to listening to your philosophy about your obesity. Often, they are open and curious about the surgery. Supporters may not share your excitement, in fact, they may appear very concerned. True supporters are concerned for you and they may even hold the belief that surgery is "drastic", but at the end of the day, they are behind you and they will support your decision.

The Critics
The critics are those people who have serious concerns about the surgery. Even though they might love you, and they may listen to you, they cannot lend their support. For whatever reason, they just cannot abide by your decision. They may or may not be teachable; it just depends on whether they are open to learning.

The Cynics
The cynics are no more than tormentors who teased the "fat kid" or befriended those who did. The cynics are bullies who are not teachable. They insist on making you feel badly about your size and your obvious lack of control. They may even laugh at your decision, so be prepared.

The Egg

As you come closer to the conclusion that weight loss surgery is for you, you may run into people who will tell you not to have surgery. They may be fat, skinny or anywhere in between. I have even heard some people go as far as to call gastric bypass surgery "mutilation". Some of them say wait on the scientists to find a cure for morbid obesity instead of jumping the gun and doing something as "drastic" as surgery. For these people I offer a simple challenge. Would they be willing to hold on to a simple egg until science finds a cure for morbid obesity? They would have to carry this egg all the times, while at work, at play, while sleeping and even having sex. Surely an egg can't be that bad to carry around, it only weighs a little, even less than a pound. If they were able to carry this egg for a week that would be notable, and if they were able to carry it for a year, that should break a record, but my guess is that they probably can't carry a simple egg for a whole day, just 24 hours. This is the interesting part. This same person who can't carry an egg for a day, is asking you to carry around over 100 extra pounds, the equivalent of about 500 or 600 eggs, for a lifetime (or at least until science can come up with the cause and cure for morbid obesity). Here's a tip for you, when dealing with the cynics in your life, think about the egg.

Before approaching others, make sure you've done your homework. Both the supporters and the critics are going to have questions for you and you want to be prepared. Read Chapter Four and do your homework first.

When, Where & How

Announcing, "I want to have weight loss surgery" at the dinner table might not work for everyone. I suggest approaching the supporters first one on one. If you don't have any supporters on your list, you will need to find one. There's a support group somewhere and I am confident that you will find a supporter even if it means finding an Internet support group.

Arrange a meeting with your supporter so that you have time to talk and some privacy to discuss your desire to have weight loss surgery. If you are close enough to the supporter, share your mental and physical burdens. Let them know that they are more than you want to deal with and also share the diets you've tried. You may want to share some of the negative feelings you've experienced about being morbidly obese. And if you think that obesity is not your fault, share that as well. If the supporter knows nothing about weight loss surgery, be prepared to share all about the surgery including how it works and what it means. Most supporters will ask questions, but I suggest that you try to cover all the information and ask them

> *Without studying and doing your homework, you may fall into the trap that weight loss surgery is magic and as soon as you get up from the operating table you're just a few short days away from "Thin Land."*

to listen. Once you are done, then entertain their questions. If you've done your homework and you understand what you've studied, your answers will be very conversational. You'll be amazed at how much you really know. It is so important to understand as much as you can about weight loss surgery. Without studying and doing your homework, you may fall into the trap that weight loss surgery is magic and as soon as you get up from the operating table you're just a few short days away from "Thin Land."

Before ending your meeting, I want you to share your list of names with the supporter. Let them know who your others supporters are as well as who your critics and cynics are. Ask them if they are willing to be with you to provide support as you share your decision with the critics (not the cynics). You may find that you need this support when dealing with the critics. Lastly, ask them to maintain your confidence by not sharing your decision unless you give them permission. Sharing with the cynics should be prohibited.

Be very careful how you approach the critics. Be aware of the meeting time and place. You want to have enough time and proper privacy. If sharing that weight loss surgery is your desire is too much, engage them in a conversation about your struggle with morbid obesity. If that is too much, you may want to take a supporter along and have them share what you've been going through. These meetings can be very emotional. The critics, like the supporters are concerned about you and your health. My mother was a critic turned supporter. It's important to realize that critics can turn into supporters. If your critic does not turn into a supporter, this is all right. As with the supporters, you want your critics to maintain confidence by not sharing your decision unless you give them permission.

This may sound harsh, but I wouldn't give a cynic the time of day. If they eventually find out about your desire to have surgery and they approach you, get a sense of whether they are a critic or a true cynic. If they are a cynic, tell them "I do not want to talk to you about this" and walk away. The cynic does not care about you or your health. Their objective is to ridicule you and make you feel badly about your decision as well as your morbid obesity. Do not try to teach a cynic. I repeat, do not try to teach a cynic. It's a useless exercise that will end in frustration and exhaustion not to mention the negativity that you will invite into your life.

Your Physician (PCP)

If your physician is a supporter, this is great! If he (or she) is a critic, try to teach them. If your physician is a cynic, change doctors immediately.

Get your insurance book and start looking over the list. Call each doctor and ask them if they are willing to work with a morbidly obese client. That's what I did. I had a critic/cynic primary care physician (PCP). I am a nurse and I shared my desire to have weight loss surgery and she told me "You didn't put that weight on overnight and it's not going to come off overnight". First of all, I didn't think it would come off overnight! If she had understood anything about weight loss surgery, she would have known that the weight comes off over a 24-month period. Do you consider two years overnight? That's a long night isn't it? Instead of fighting with this woman, I harkened back to the lessons from my fat kid years and I exercised some emotional control. I nodded and listened to her tell me that I should push myself away from the table, go to the gym and talk to a counselor. Perhaps her advice was good, but I had pushed myself away from the table, I was too big to "move right" and I didn't need a counselor. I needed surgery. That was the last day I ever saw her. One week later I requested a copy of my medical file in writing and moved on to the next doctor who was a supporter. You do not have to leave a practice formally, just request your records from the office manager, not the doctor. The office will have you sign a medical release form and in some cases pay a small copying fee. Unfortunately, there are too many physician critics and cynics. But life goes on...

Chapter Four

"I am ready, I want my life back. My BMI is 62.4, and I have high blood pressure, sleep apnea, joint pain and shortness of breath. I am still young (43), and I am not able to do the things I love to do, I want to do them again. My job is at stake because of mobility, as is my life in general."

"I was denied by the Medical Director from my insurance group. He stated that I need to contact my PCP and go over alternative methods of weight loss. What a joke. I called my insurance company and they made me feel a lot better, they told me to get copies of everything supporting my case and send it directly to them. More waiting."

"There are people out there that don't believe in GOD. God is watching over me big time. PTL."

"I can't describe my feeling right now except to say the light at the end of the tunnel is not a train..."

"I was not able be to have my surgery laparoscopically due to too many surgeries. That was a disappointment. I have gone full steam ahead and then I started taking a few steps back, with just three days to go I got a little nervous."

"I continue to receive comments on how good I look and I have been told by my father the greatest change he sees is my attitude. My will to live is back and my life is getting better every day. I still continue to feel like any day I am going to wake up and this has all been a dream. So far so good."

Gayle Hickerson
Open DS, 10/2/2000

Knowledge Overcomes Fear

Your Surgical Options

Chances are, if you are reading this far, you are curious about weight loss surgery. It is important for you to understand what weight loss surgery is and what it does. You need to take the time to learn and understand weight loss surgery. Knowledge overcomes fear (and false propaganda) about weight loss surgery. In this chapter, I am going to provide an outline of each basic weight loss surgery offered today. All of the options are safe and effective. Your final decision about which surgery you select is ultimately yours. Spend some time understanding each surgery. I also suggest that you meet other people who have had the surgery. They will be an invaluable reference for you. In the Appendix section, I have included the web addresses of some good on-line support groups for each surgery offered today. The wonderful support communities are open about sharing their stories with you.

I'll start with a small history lesson and then a basic anatomy lesson and then we'll get into understanding the surgeries.

History Lesson 101

The history of weight loss surgery began as an observation actually. Doctors did not set out on a path to find a treatment for morbid obesity. What happened is that stomach and intestinal cancer patients who had parts of the stomach and or intestine removed lost a considerable amount of weight and it was thought that if part of the stomach or intestine were removed, weight loss would occur. The same thought pattern existed for the surgical pioneers who, in a sense, invented bypass surgery for weight loss. If the stomach were smaller, people couldn't eat as much and if food went through less of the intestine, less food would be absorbed. Like anything new, the first version is usually not the best version, it's experimental and requires updating or upgrading. The earlier gastric bypass surgeries were difficult for the patients and many of them spent weeks and months in intensive care and many died. The surgeons did not know how much of the stomach to alter, and they didn't know how much intestine or even which part of the intestine was best to bypass. So the first decade or so, people who had bypass surgery had it pretty rough and the term "intestinal bypass" got a bad wrap. But over the past decade, the entire evolution of gastric bypass surgery has grown into a very knowledgeable area of medicine known as bariatric surgery. Today, we know so much more and the mortality rate for bariatric surgery is less than 1%. This is the same mortality rate for almost any major surgery when you factor in that the person being operated on is morbidly obese. Intensive care stays and food intolerances have decreased sharply and significantly. The rate of infection and the length of hospital stay have decreased significantly thanks to the advancements of minimally invasive surgical techniques. My own surgery was done on an outpatient basis! Because the science of bariatric surgery is only 30-40 years old, many people know someone who may have suffered as a result of the early years. Their experiences have scared many people because they don't know that things have improved greatly. We should never forget the past, but we can't live there either. Like all medical advances, they start as experimental, but end up as accepted standards of practice. Today, the National Institute of Health recommends bariatric surgery as the treatment of choice and medically necessary care for those with morbid obesity.

Anatomy Lesson 101

Food goes into the mouth, down the esophagus and into the stomach. When food leaves the stomach, it enters the small intestine. The small intestine is about 20 feet long. It has three distinct parts. The first part is called the duodenum (which is less than a foot long), the next section is the jejunum and the last part is the ileum. After food moves through the small intestine, it enters and travels through the large intestine, which is also known as the colon and then exits the body. (See the diagram)

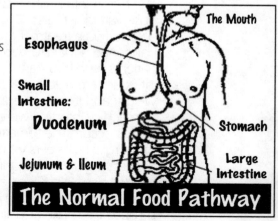

The Normal Food Pathway

Weight loss surgery or gastric bypass surgery involves two parts: the stomach and the small intestine. Remember that the small intestine has three parts. When weight loss surgery involves the stomach only and not the small intestine, this is called gastroplasty. Gastroplasty is not gastric bypass surgery, but all gastric bypass surgeries include gastroplasty because the stomach is changed or altered. I do want to point out that gastroplasty surgery is also known as "stomach stapling" (I hate that term). Genetically predisposed morbidly obese people who have had gastroplasty surgery (and not gastric bypass) tend to regain their weight. It is for this reason that I strongly urge morbidly obese people to have gastric bypass surgery and not just gastroplasty. Gastroplasty does have a place and I think it works best for the people who are 70 to 80 pounds overweight. I also think it works for people who have not had a lifetime struggle with obesity, but they gained a significant amount of weight after a "life event" like having children. These people may not have a genetic predisposition for obesity or even morbid obesity. For whatever reason, they seemed to gain weight and they need help to get the 70 to 80 pounds off and gastroplasty may be the answer for them.

One Goal Three Surgeries

There are three basic gastric bypass or weight loss surgeries performed today. Despite what titles the surgeries have been given, there are only three basic surgeries. They are: the Billroth II Loop Bypass (Billroth II), the Roux-en-Y (RNY) Gastric Bypass and the Duodenal Diversion (or Duodenal Switch, DS). Before I explain these three surgeries, I want you to know that surgical advancements in the area of laparoscopic surgery are available and all three of these gastric bypass surgeries can be done with a minimally invasive approach. This means that you do not have to have a full incision. With laparoscopic surgery, small pencil size tools are used to perform the surgery. Five to six very small incisions or "port hole" sites are used. The abdomen is "expanded" with gas. The tools have small cameras on the end of them and the surgeon is able to do the surgery by viewing your insides on a TV-like monitor. This type of surgery greatly reduces the recovery time and the time you will spend in the hospital. My surgery was done outpatient and I left the hospital on the same day of my surgery. Laparascopic surgery is an amazing advancement. At the writing of this book, there are only a handful of high-volume laparascopic gastric bypass surgeons in the country, but I strongly suspect that in time this will become more commonplace as more surgeons are trained in the art of using laparascopic tools. Open incisions will still be performed because not everyone is a candidate for laparascopic surgery. You will have to have a consult with the surgeon to see if there are reasons that you would not qualify for laparascopic abdominal surgery. The open incision approach for gastric bypass surgery involves a 4 to 12 inch incision. The incision can be horizontal (going east to west) or vertical (going north to south). The size and direction of the incision depends on your body, your surgeon and which surgery you choose.

All three gastric bypass surgeries alter the size and shape of the stomach. Some surgeons use staples and others use sutures or stitches. It just depends on your surgeon and their technique. The normal stomach is about the size of two fists. It is shaped sort of like a kidney bean and when stretched, it can hold anywhere from 1.5 to 4 quarts.

Each of the three surgeries alters the food pathway. Recall that food goes from the stomach to the duodenum then to the jejunum. After gastric bypass surgery, food will no longer see the duodenum. Instead, food will travel from the stomach to the jejunum. It is the duodenum that is being bypassed.

To help you better understand all three surgeries, I will first cover what changes happen to the stomach. This is the gastroplasty part of the surgery.

The New Stomach

The Normal Stomach

First, take a good look at the normal stomach. (See the diagram). The stomach will be made smaller using staples or stitches.

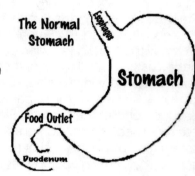

The Billroth II Stomach

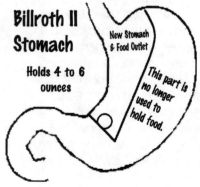

The stomach is narrowed and takes on the shape of a tube instead of the kidney shape. The new stomach can hold four to six ounces. The stomach is cut in such a way that stretching is minimized. A new food outlet is created at the end of the new stomach. Notice the old and the new food outlets in the diagram.

The RNY Stomach

The "typical" RNY stomach is cut on a diagonal angle close to the esophagus. The stomach will hold one but no more than two ounces. This is about the size of your thumb. A new food outlet is created in the new stomach. Notice the old and the new food outlets in the diagram.

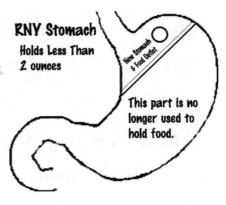

RNY Stomach

Holds Less Than 2 ounces

New Stomach & Food Outlet

This part is no longer used to hold food.

The DS Stomach

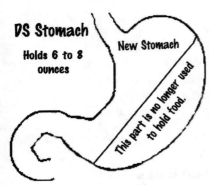

DS Stomach

Holds 6 to 8 ounces

New Stomach

This part is no longer used to hold food.

The Duodenal Switch stomach is the largest of the three gastric surgeries. It usually holds six to eight ounces. It is cut along a diagonal border as well, but unlike the Billroth II or RNY stomach, a new food outlet is not created because the DS uses the existing food outlet. See the diagram.

Keep in mind that each surgeon has their own preferences and they don't have to follow any set rules. The larger the size of the stomach, the more food it can hold and the more natural or normal your eating patterns. There is less occurrence of nausea problems with a larger stomach. A year after surgery though, more normal eating patterns start to resume even with a one ounce stomach. The size of your stomach should be discussed with your doctor and you should have the right to ask for what you want. I recommend that you draw a kidney shaped stomach and ask your surgeon to draw on it so that you will see what the new shape of your stomach will look like. This way you know before surgery what your stomach will hold. If you want a larger stomach or a smaller stomach, be prepared to discuss this with your surgeon. Be aware that the size of your stomach does not determine how much weight you will lose or how fast you will lose weight. This is determined by several factors, we'll talk about that later. Regardless of the size or shape of your new stomach, one thing is certain. You will eat less, much less than before.

Just in case you are wondering what happens to the old stomach and the old food outlet, it stays in the body. They still have a function.

In the case of the Billroth II and the RNY, the old food outlet is still connected to the duodenum. I'll explain more about that later on. For now, let's move on to the second part of the gastric bypass surgery.

The New Plumbing - The Actual Bypass

The Normal Food Pathway

Before studying the new food pathway, take a minute to go back and look at the normal anatomy and food pathway. The graphic that I used under "Anatomy 101" shows that the small intestine folds back and forth in the abdominal cavity. I want you to think of the food pathway as one long tube that extends from the mouth all the way down to the colon. What I have done in the graphic below shows the food pathway as one long tube or hose. Also notice that I have listed all three parts of the small intestine. Understanding that this food pathway is really just one long hose will help you understand the different bypass surgeries.

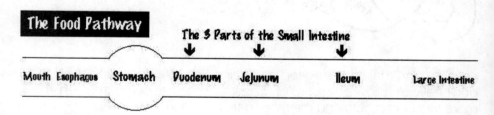

The Food Pathway

The 3 Parts of the Small Intestine

Mouth Esophagus Stomach Duodenum Jejunum Ileum Large Intestine

The NEW Food Pathway

In Chapter Two, I explained that for the genetically predisposed morbidly obese person, something goes crazy when food hits the duodenum. The objective or goal of the bypass part of the surgery is to reroute (or bypass) the duodenum so that food never, ever sees the duodenum ever again. I am convinced that this is the part of the genetically predisposed morbidly obese person's body that is not working correctly.

Each of the three surgeries has a specific way of rerouting the food pathway so that food will go from the stomach to the jejunum, bypassing the duodenum. Keep in mind as I start explaining each of the three surgeries that the jejunum is eight to ten feet long. Also keep in mind that the intestine is a very flexible hose. Think of it as a Slinky.

The Billroth II Loop Bypass

The surgeon will choose a point along the jejunum and create or "poke" a new hole. Think about a water hose. If you poke a hole in the center of the hose, this is a new opening. The new food outlet created in the new stomach will be connected to this hole in the jejunum. Food will exit the new stomach and enter into this new hole in the jejunum. Food will then travel from the jejunum, to the ileum and then to the large intestine. Food will not travel backwards from the jejunum back to the duodenum because of intestinal digestive movements called peristalsis. The same movements work in the esophagus. The reason food continues to go down the esophagus and not back out of the mouth is because of peristalsis movements. To "upchuck" the food is to go against the peristaltic movements and this is abnormal. The same is true for the new opening in the jejunum. Food will not travel back into the duodenum, that would be very abnormal, and even if it did, the peristaltic movements would keep the food moving down the jejunum, to the ileum and then to the large intestine. See the diagram.

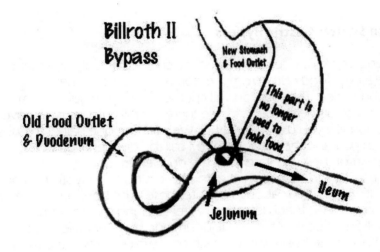

Roux-en-Y Gastric Bypass

The surgeon will find a point along the jejunum. But instead of poking a hole to create new opening, a full cut is made in the hose so that you have two hoses and not just one. Think about that water hose again. If you cut the hose in two you now have two hoses. We'll call one hose the duodenal half and we will call the other side the jejunum half. The surgeon will take the jejunum half and connect this to the new food outlet in the new stomach. Food will exit the new stomach and enter into the jejunum. Food will then travel from the jejunum, to the ileum and then to the large intestine. Further down the jejunum the surgeon will poke a hole. The other hose, the duodenal half is connected to this new hole further down the jejunum. This new connection gives the shape of the letter Y, hence the name Roux-en-Y. See the diagram.

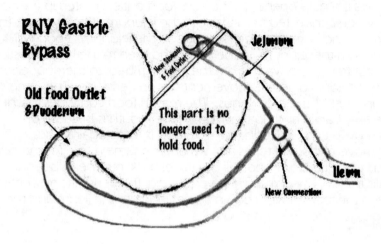

Duodenal Switch Gastric Bypass

Remember that the duodenal switch stomach was the only one that did not create a new food outlet from the stomach because it uses the existing food outlet. The surgeon will cut the neck of the duodenum right at the base of the stomach. Since there is a full cut, you now have two hoses, just like you did in the RNY. We'll call the one half of the hose the stomach part and the other half we'll call the duodenal part. The duodenal part of the hose starts with the duodenum and ends at the large intestine. The duodenal end of the hose is completely stitched or stapled shut. Again, think about the water hose. The hose has one end stitched and one end that is left open. After stitching this end shut, the surgeon will find a point along the jejunum and make another full cut. Now you have three hoses: the stomach part, which starts at the mouth and ends at the stomach, the duodenal part, which starts at the duodenum and ends at some point in the jejunum and lastly the jejunum part, which starts at some point in the jejunum and ends at the colon. The jejunum part is then connected to the food outlet in the stomach. I can also say it in this way. The top of the jejunum part (hose number three) is sewn or connected to the end of the stomach part (hose number one). This is done so that food will exit the stomach and enter into the jejunum. Food will then travel from the jejunum to the ileum and then to the large intestine. Also like the RNY, there is still that open end of the duodenal part of the hose, remember that the one end of the hose is stitched shut. Further down the jejunum the surgeon will poke a hole. The open end of the hose, the duodenal part is connected to this new hole further down the jejunum. (See the diagram.)

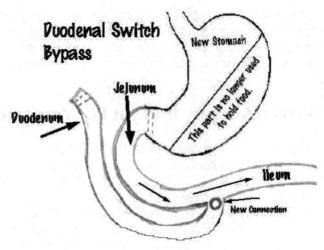

Duodenal Switch Bypass

New Stomach

Jejunum

Duodenum

This part is no longer used to hold food.

Ileum

New Connection

Summary

Billroth II	One cut in the stomach Two new holes: one in new stomach and one in the jejunum
RNY	Two cuts: one in the stomach and in the jejunum Two new holes: one in the stomach and one in the jejunum
DS	Three cuts: the first in the stomach, the second at the neck of the duodenum and the third in the jejunum One new hole in the jejunum

If this is all too confusing for you, just know that in any of the three surgeries, food will never, ever again see the duodenum and that is the objective or goal of the bypass.

Anatomy Lesson 102

Here's another small anatomy lesson. I didn't show it in any of the diagrams, but there's a tiny tube or duct that goes from the liver, pancreas and the gall bladder to the duodenum. This is called the common bile duct. Bile and digestive enzymes are created in the liver, gall bladder and pancreas. They enter the small intestine at the level of the duodenum. For this reason (and more) the stomach and the duodenum are all left intact and not thrown out. Even though food no longer travels down the duodenal pathway, those digestive juices still travel down the pathway and the digestive juices meet up with the food again in the jejunum. This digestive process allows food to still break down naturally.

To minimize any problems associated with the gall bladder, about half of the bariatric surgeons will remove the gall bladder at the time they do the gastric bypass or they will have the patient take medication (bile salts) for a few weeks or months after surgery to prevent gall bladder problems.

Which Surgery Is Right For You

Each surgeon fiercely defends his or her own surgery. Each of the three surgeries has its risks and potential complications. All of the surgeries offer the same great weight loss outcome. There is a greater than 99% chance that you will lose over half or more of your excess body weight and keep it off as long as you maintain reasonable eating and exercise. There is no denying that the results with gastric bypass surgery are stellar. I have chosen to not enter into the ongoing debates over which surgery is best because it is terribly subjective. Everybody has an opinion, but the fact is that the evolution of gastric bypass will continue with medical and surgical advances.

To date, the most common of the three surgeries is the open RNY, but this is because it has been performed the longest and only a small number of surgeons have mastered the technique of laparascopic surgery giving them the skills to correctly perform minimally invasive videoscopic surgery. Contrary to the cynics and the critics, the Duodenal Switch is not the old jejunum-ileum (JI) intestinal bypass and the Billroth II Loop Bypass is not the old Mason loop bypass. Some bariatric surgeons complain that the laparascopic surgery is not as "good" as the open surgery. The reason I am pointing this out is because there are some zealous critics who complain about the newer surgeries and laparascopic techniques. For their own reasons, they are not open to grow with the bariatric industry. I have met hundreds of people who have had every kind of surgery outlined in this chapter. Very few have experienced any complications and all of them report that they would have their surgery again in a heartbeat.

We can't forget the past, but we can't live it either. In the Appendix section, I have included the web addresses of some good on-line support groups for each surgery offered today. The wonderful support communities are open about sharing their stories with you. Whichever surgery you choose, I believe you will be satisfied with the outcome. For myself and many others, the risks of remaining morbidly obese far outweighed the risks of surgery.

The Benefits

Permanent Weight Loss
Any diet will help you lose weight, but the chance of keeping it off is almost impossible.

Turn Around of the Co-morbidities & Complications
If you have sleep apnea, type two diabetes, hypertension or joint pain, many or most people report no longer having these problems after the weight is down.

Improved Mental Outlook
The emotional burdens associated with morbid obesity are many. When you are no longer morbidly obese, you will still have emotional burdens, this surgery does not get rid of all of your stress, but it does improve your mental outlook.

Improved Mortality Rate
Sadly, morbid obesity cuts away at your chance of living a long healthy life. When the weight is down, your chance for a normal mortality is greatly improved.

The Surgical Risks

Infection (of any type)
Anytime the body is cut open, there is a risk of infection. There is also a risk of contracting an infection whenever you are admitted to the hospital. Any surgery carries the risk of infection. Wound care is very important.

Wound Dehiscence
This means that the wound can re-open after surgery. This risk increases if your abdomen is very large. The risk of the wound reopening with laparascopic surgery is very small because the incisions are tiny.

Incision Hernia
When the wound heals, the muscles underneath the skin knit back together. If the underlying muscle does not knit back together properly, a hernia will develop. Hernias are repairable and are not life threatening. The chance of incision hernias are very rare with laparascopic surgery.

Narrowing or Constricting of the Roux Limb

The Billroth II surgery does not have a roux limb. The RNY and the DS do have a roux limb. These new limbs can narrow and constrict. If this occurs, it is correctable by surgery. The surgeon must use a tool to stretch the narrowed part of the opening. This can be done outpatient with an endoscope.

Connection Leaks

Anytime there is a new connection, there is a risk of a leak. The chances of a leak occurring are small, but they can happen within the first month of surgery. If you don't have a leak by then, it is unlikely you will develop a leak later on.

Pulmonary Embolism and Blood Clots

Whenever you are put under general anesthesia (or you are put to sleep), the blood doesn't flow as well. The blood flow is sluggish and this "slow flow" can cause the blood to thicken up. This thickening is called clot formation. Clots are dangerous, very dangerous. Because of this, some surgeons will have you on blood thinners to prevent this problem. The longer you are under general anesthesia, the greater the risk of clot formation. When the clot travels to the lung, and stays there, it is called a pulmonary embolism. They are not always easy to detect. Usually there are some breathing problems, even if they seem small to you. For this reason, coughing and deep breathing exercises are very important after surgery. Walking is also important. The longer you stay down, the higher your risk of clot formation. The Billroth II surgery offers the great advantage of being under anesthesia less than an hour, sometimes this procedure can be done in less than 30 minutes. Getting up to walk after surgery is relatively easy to do with laparascopic surgery. The advantage of laparascopic surgery is that the incisions are so small, there is much less pain post-op.

Malnutrition

Food is still being absorbed, but you are taking in less food. The food intake is not being absorbed the same as it was before surgery because the duodenum has been bypassed. For this reason, you must monitor your intake and take vitamins the rest of your life. I will talk more about this later on.

Bile Reflux, Ulcers & Cancer

You may remember that the bile, liver and pancreatic enzymes still enter the duodenum and travel down that pathway even though food does not. There is a small chance that these digestive juices can irritate the lining of the intestine because it no longer mixes with food until later on in the intestine. In addition, the Billroth II Loop Bypass has a small risk associated with these digestive juices entering the new stomach. The risks are small, but they are real. In addition there's the risk for the Billroth II and the RNY surgeries that these digestive juices can travel back into the old stomach since the food outlet is kept intact. The DS surgery uses the existing food outlet. Again, the risks are small, but they are real. If this does occur, the symptoms are the same as any ulcer symptoms, which are burning and gastric irritation. Because this is a risk, you may want to have an annual endoscopy. Like any other regular test whether it be a colonoscopy, a pap smear or a mammogram, you are using them to catch a problem before it gets out of control. The endoscopy test is one where a tube goes down the throat (you are semi-conscious) and the doctor takes pictures. There is also an ultrasound test that can be done to detect gastric problems. If ulcers go untreated, and continually get worse, further damage can occur. Generally speaking, you would have caught the ulcer at an early stage due to the symptoms of an ulcer. Acid-induced ulcers are treated medically with antacids, acid controllers and proton acid pump inhibitors.

Don't panic if you have gastric ulcers. It is very important to point out that 99% of all ulcers are NOT caused by acid as it was once believed. Ninety-nine percent of ulcers are caused by a bacteria called H-pylori. This bacteria can be killed with a simple broad spectrum antibiotic. To learn more about H-pylori and ulcers, you can go to the information website about ulcers from the Center for Disease Control at http://www.cdc.gov/ulcer or you can read more about it at the Foundation for H-pylori at http://www.helico.com.

Death
The risk of dying due to this surgery is far less than 1%. But death is a reality. Most of the deaths are caused by a pulmonary embolism followed by infections or uncontrolled bleeding. It is rare, but it has happened. I can't emphasize enough that all surgery has the risk of death.

Conversions, Revisions & Reversals...

Just in case science ever comes up with a magic genetic fix, all of the surgeries can be reversed. The gastroplasty part of the surgery can be reversed, but I'm not sure how well the stomach will "work" after being altered (meaning stapled and cut). The bypass portion for the Billroth II is the easiest to reverse since there is no full intestinal cut.

In addition, all of the surgeries can be revised or updated. In some cases the stomach may need to be altered again or the amount of small intestine that is bypassed may need to be altered. If too much weight is lost or not enough weight is lost, a revision is an option for all three surgeries.

For those people who elect to have gastroplasty without gastric bypass, conversion to a full gastric bypass is possible and quite common.

In June, 2001, the FDA approved a device for gastroplasty that does not involve any staples or cutting of the stomach. The procedure can be done laparoscopically. It is called the LAP-BAND. You can learn more about this gastroplasty surgery and the LAP-BAND device at: http://www.bioenterics.com/us/products/lapband/index.html

Chapter Five

"This surgery has given me the freedom to focus my attention on things more important than my outward appearance."

"Gone are those days of watching late-night infomercials, wondering "could this be the one that works?""

"Sometimes it takes getting to the point of quiet desperation before one looks for solutions outside themselves. Where are you?"

"Surgery for me, was an anxious experience, a reality check, and a blessing which took months to appreciate."

"Many people ask me how my surgical experience was. I realize for many, it is a scary time, but I truly went into this experience, with the full expectation that God would protect me through this process, because His hand was at work from the day He heard my prayers and approved my insurance request."

"As I lost weight, I began looking forward to tomorrow. I began taking chances in my personal and professional life, and I found myself reclaiming the right to walk tall in this society, without excuse, like everyone else."

Deana Barbosa
http://www.geocities.com/Indiroo_28/Home_2.html
Laparascopic RNY, 8/9/1999

Am I A Candidate For Obesity Surgery?

Obesity Facts...

- The U.S. Census Bureau estimates that there are about 58 million obese adults in America: 26 million men and 32 million women.
- Obesity increased by 9 percent among women and men ages 20 to 74 between 1960 and 1991.
- One third (33.4%) of American adults are estimated to be obese.
- Maintaining weight loss is exceedingly difficult for the morbidly obese. Most people regain as much as two-thirds of weight lost within one year and regain all of it and then some within five years.

Am I A Candidate For Bariatric Surgery?

This all depends on whom you ask. If you are asking your PCP, you will get one answer. If you are asking the bariatric surgeon, you will get another answer. There are nationally recognized standards established by the National Institute of Health and Milliman & Robertson, which is a nationally recognized source for establishing medical necessity for the insurance industry. Still, the insurance carrier will have its own set of standards that they will use to judge whether or not you are "worthy" of having bariatric surgery.

The PCP

In Chapter Three, I addressed dealing with your primary care physician (PCP). Most surgeons will require a referral from your PCP. The job of the surgeon usually begins and ends with surgery. A surgeon works with the PCP, but the surgeon is not your PCP. Both the PCP and the surgeon are both doctors, but their roles are very different. There are still too many PCP's who are critics and cynics and they respond negatively to the idea of weight loss surgery. Despite the fact that the nationally recognized protocol for morbid obesity is surgical treatment and that surgical intervention is the only treatment option that shows any long term success for overcoming morbid obesity, they hold on to the belief system that bariatric surgery is something they cannot agree to. If this is your PCP, you need to switch. Fortunately, many other primary care physicians are very supportive. If you have a supportive and knowledgeable PCP, he or she will probably defer to the national guidelines and standards established by the National Institute of Health.

The Surgeon

Each bariatric surgeon will have his or her own set of criteria as well. Most bariatric surgeons will not perform gastric bypass surgery on you if you are less than 80 or 100 pounds overweight. Another measure that is used to indicate morbid obesity is the body mass index or BMI. Most bariatric surgeons require that your BMI be at least 35. The relationship with the surgeon will often begin with a referral, even if it's a self-referral. The surgeon should offer something in writing that outlines their criteria for being a surgical candidate. It is unlikely that the bariatric surgeon will go against the national guidelines and standards established by the National Institute of Health, The American Society for Bariatric Surgery guidelines or the guidelines established by Milliman & Robertson. Some surgeons will have even more stringent guidelines for being a surgical candidate.

My Surgeon's Criteria

To illustrate the additional criteria that a surgeon may require for patient selection, I have included the criteria set by my surgeon.
- A well functioning Email address that can accept "attachments"
- Between age 16 and 55
- A BMI of 40 kg/m2 or above, or a BMI of 35 to 40 with a co-morbidity
- A body weight no more than 350 lbs
- Patients must presently be working, either in or out of the home
- No history of previous obesity surgery
- No history of major abdominal surgery
- No history of alcohol abuse or drug use
- The patient must show evidence of a stable family structure and have the documented support of their immediate family

- The patient must have a personal physician who will:
  - Support the patient for Gastric Bypass
  - Perform a detailed preoperative evaluation
  - Will actively follow the patient after the operation with the surgeon
- No history of major psychiatric illness
- If the patient has a history of depression, the patient and his or her psychiatrist must have a plan in place with their psychiatrist for the diagnosis and management of depression postoperatively.
- No history of recent Prednisone therapy, Systemic Lupus Erythematosis (SLE), Rheumatoid Arthritis or other collagen vascular disease.
- Documented commitment to participate in a postoperative exercise program.
- Documented commitment to maintain yearly long-term follow-up with the surgeon to decrease the risks of vitamin, mineral and other nutritional deficiencies.

The ASBS

There is an association for bariatric surgeons. It is the American Society for Bariatric Surgery (ASBS). Not all bariatric surgeons are members of the ASBS. The ASBS has published a paper that outlines a set of patient selection criteria (www.asbs.org). They state that the option of surgical treatment should be offered to patients who are morbidly obese, well informed, motivated, and have accepted the operative risks. The patient should be able to participate in treatment and long-term follow-up. Patients that are mentally ill may not be able to offer an informed consent and cooperation with long-term follow-up, therefore they may need to be excluded. The decision to elect surgical treatment requires an assessment of the risk and benefit in each case. Functional impairments associated with obesity are also important deciding factors for surgical treatment.

The patients who have a BMI that exceeds 40 are potential candidates for surgery if they strongly desire substantial weight loss, because morbid obesity impairs the quality of life. They must clearly and realistically understand how their life may change after the operation.

In certain circumstances, less morbidly obese patients who have a BMI between 35 and 40 may also be considered for surgery. Included in this category are patients with high-risk co-morbid conditions such as life threatening cardiopulmonary problems. Other possible indications include obesity-induced physical problems that are interfering with their lifestyle, like the ability to work and earn a living.

The Insurer

While the medical professional, the PCP and the surgeon readily default to the national guidelines, the insurance company can and will make up their own guidelines to qualify or disqualify you. It is sad, but many insurance companies make the guidelines so stringent that almost no morbidly obese person will qualify. It should be against the law. The nationally recognized insurance industry standard is Milliman & Robertson, but the insurance industry is under no jurisdiction to follow these guidelines. They are able to make up their own rules. I have devoted an entire chapter to dealing with the insurance company. My fight with my insurance company was awful!

Blue Cross Blue Shield Of North Carolina

Blue Cross Blue Shield of North Carolina published its weight loss surgery guidelines in The Corporate Medical Policy on Surgery for Morbid Obesity. It states that surgery for morbid obesity is covered when ALL of the following criteria are met.

- When obesity has been present for at least five years and non-surgical methods of accomplishing weight reduction under a physician's supervision have failed.
- The patient must be at least 100% overweight.
- The patient must be 50% or 100 pounds over weight, whichever is greater. In addition, the excess weight must be associated with at least one of the following problems:
    - The obesity interferes with daily function to the extent that performance is significantly curtailed (i.e., impending job loss or job loss with documented disability).
    - The obesity causes incapacitating physical trauma as documented by the medical history records including x-ray findings and other diagnostic test results.
    - There is significant respiratory insufficiency documented by respiratory function studies, blood gases, etc.
    - There is significant circulatory insufficiency documented by objective measurements.
    - There is documentation that the management of primary diseases such as arteriosclerosis, diabetes, heart disease, etc., is complicated by the obesity.
- The patient has no specifically correctable cause for the obesity, e.g., an endocrine disorder
- Patient has achieved full growth.

The National Institute of Health (NIH)

First Federal Guidelines, 1998

The first federal obesity clinical guidelines were released in 1998. In this report, weight loss surgery is an option for carefully selected patients with clinically severe obesity. Clinically severe obesity was defined as a BMI of $\geq$ 40 or BMI of $\geq$35 with coexisting co-morbid conditions. The surgical treatment would be appropriate when less invasive methods of weight loss had been tried and failed and the patient is at high risk for obesity-associated illness. The guidelines also call for lifelong medical surveillance after surgery is a necessity.

The press release is printed in the Appendix along with the web site address and information for obtaining the 282-page landmark study on obesity.

NIH Consensus Statement, 1991

The patient selection criteria established by the National Institute of Health's Consensus Development Conference in March of 1991, states that there is insufficient data on which to base recommendations for patient selection using objective clinical features alone. A decision to surgically treat morbid obesity requires assessing the risk-benefit ratio in each case. Those patients judged by experienced clinicians to have a low probability of success with nonsurgical measures, as demonstrated for example by failures in established weight control programs or reluctance by the patient to enter such a program, may be considered for surgery.

A gastric bypass procedure should be considered only for well-informed and motivated patients who accept and understand the operative risks. The patient should be able to participate in treatment and long-term follow-up.

The patient's BMI should exceed 40 and the potential candidates for surgery should strongly desire substantial weight loss, because obesity severely impairs their quality of life. They must clearly and realistically understand how their life may change after operation.

In certain instances obese patients with a BMI of 35 should also be considered for surgery. Included in this category are patients with high-risk co-morbid conditions such as life-threatening cardiopulmonary problems or severe diabetes mellitus. Other possible indications for patients with a BMI between 35-40 include obesity-induced physical problems interfering with their lifestyle.

Children and adolescents have not been sufficiently studied to allow a recommendation for surgery, even in the face of a BMI over 40.

Milliman & Robertson

The obesity treatment guidelines from Milliman and Robertson for gastric bypass surgery for clinically severe obesity state that the patient must be at least 100 pounds over the ideal weight as defined by the Metropolitan Life tables (see Appendix) or the patient must have a body mass index exceeding 40. If the body mass index is 35, they must present with a clinically serious condition like obesity hypoventilation, sleep apnea, diabetes, hypertension, cardiomyopathy or musculoskeletal dysfunction. The patient must show that they have failed to lose weight significantly or has regained weight despite compliance with a multidisciplinary non-surgical programs including a low or very low calorie diet, supervised exercise, behavior modification and support. The patient should not have any correctable cause for obesity like an endocrine disorder. The patient must be full-grown and have reached full growth (this would exclude children). The patient should be treated in a surgical program with experience in obesity surgery, including, not only surgeons experienced with gastric bypass, but also a multidisciplinary approach including all of the following: preoperative medical consultation and approval, preoperative psychiatric consultation and approval, nutritional counseling, exercise counseling, psychological counseling and support group discussions.

Am I A Candidate or Not?

Again, it depends on whom you ask. Your answer will probably start with your insurance company if you want the insurance company to pay for the surgery. If you are paying for the surgery yourself, then you will start with the surgeon's requirements. Because the surgeon will want to have your PCP do follow-up, you will also need to meet the criteria for your PCP.

Potential Surgical Qualifications Checklist

Qualification	Yes	No	N/A
Are you morbidly obese?			
Are you well informed?			
Are you motivated?			
Have you accepted the operative risks?			

Qualification	Yes	No	N/A
Are you able to participate in treatment?			
Are you able to participate in long-term follow-up?			
Do you think that the benefits for surgery outweigh the risks?			
Do you have any functional impairment associated with obesity?			
Does your BMI exceed 40?			
Do you strongly desire substantial weight loss?			
Has obesity impaired your quality of life?			
Do you clearly and realistically understand how your life may change after the operation?			
Is your BMI over 35 with high-risk co-morbid conditions such as life threatening cardiopulmonary problems?			
Do you have obesity-induced physical problems that is interfering with your lifestyle?			
Have you been obese for at least five years?			
Have you tried non-surgical methods of accomplishing weight reduction under a physician's supervision and have failed?			
Are you at least 100% overweight?			
Are you 50% or 100 pounds over weight, whichever is greater?			
Does obesity interfere with your daily function to the extent that performance is significantly curtailed?			
Does obesity causes incapacitating physical trauma as documented by the medical history records including x-ray findings and other diagnostic test results?			
Is there significant respiratory insufficiency documented by respiratory function studies and blood gases?			

Qualification	Yes	No	N/A
Is there significant circulatory insufficiency documented by objective measurements?			
Is there documentation that the management of primary diseases such as arteriosclerosis, diabetes and heart disease are complicated by the obesity?			
Do you have a specific correctable cause for the obesity like an endocrine disorder?			
Have you achieved full growth? Are you over adolescent age?			
Are you at high risk for obesity-associated illness?			
Are you wiling to participate in lifelong medical surveillance after surgery?			
Do you have obesity hypoventilation, sleep apnea, diabetes, hypertension, cardiomyopathy or musculoskeletal dysfunction?			
Have you failed to lose weight significantly or have you regained weight despite compliance with a multidisciplinary non-surgical programs including a low or very low calorie diet, supervised exercise, behavior modification and support?			
Have you had a surgeon's preoperative medical consultation and approval?			
Have you had a preoperative psychiatric consultation and approval?			
Have you had any nutritional counseling?			
Have you had any exercise counseling?			
Have you had any psychological counseling?			
Have you participated in any support group discussions?			

Chapter Six

"I was the chubby child who was picked last for the recess games. I was the overweight teenager who didn't date in high school or go to prom. I was the obese college student who wasn't invited to the parties. I was the morbidly obese professional woman who struggled to prove myself in the workplace. My entire life, I have been overweight. I always kept a smile on my face and seemed happy as can be, trying not to let the world around me see me dying inside."

"I was very successful at the other things that I did. So why couldn't I lose weight? I tried and tried to lose weight for almost twenty years. I was at the end of my rope, weighing in at 298 pounds at 28 years old."

"I had weight loss surgery, and it has been a wonderful and scary transition for me ever since. My life has completely changed, and I have been reborn! I have been bungee jumping, white water rafting, hiking, camping, and doing all of the wonderful things that life has to offer. People say that I glow with happiness. I have never been happier in my life."

Mellissa Barcelo
http://www.duodenalswitch.com/Patients/Mellissa/mellissa.html
Open DS, 1/14/1998

Selecting Your Surgeon

Did You Know There Are Over 700 Bariatric Surgeons?

There are over 700 bariatric surgeons in the America. Finding a surgeon in your state is easy to do if you have Internet access. The Association for Morbid Obesity Support at http://www.obesityhelp.com is a great place to start. There's a database of bariatric surgeons that you can search by state or last name.

I understand that for many readers, your choice of a bariatric surgeon will be dictated by your insurance carrier. Your insurance coverage may limit your choice of a surgeon. If this is the case, you can still start your search at obesityhelp.com, but you will also need to see if the bariatric surgeon is on your insurance list.

Your choice of surgeon may also be narrowed if you want laparascopic surgery. As of the writing of this book, there are less than 50 laparascopic gastric bypass surgeons, but this number is growing rapidly. If you want a surgeon who specializes in weight loss surgery exclusively, your choice will be narrowed to 200 surgeons. If you want one of the newer bariatric surgeries like the Billroth II or the Duodenal Switch, your choice will be limited to less than 25 high-volume laparascopic bariatric surgeons.

Today, the landslide majority of surgeons are trained and qualified to perform the open Roux-en-Y gastric bypass procedure.

I strongly suggest that whichever surgeon you choose, please attend their support group meetings either on-line or in person. A surgeon's best advertisement are their previous patient's personal experiences. If the surgeon does not have an active support group or if they cannot provide you with the names of some previous patients, this could be a potential red warning flag of caution. Another service that obesityhelp.com offers is a list of patient comments about their experience with the surgeon.

You will find that the Internet is an invaluable resource for you in your weight loss surgery journey.

I also suggest that you ask the office for an information packet. Each surgeon will have his or her own criteria for patient selection. The surgeon should be able to mail you information or provide you with a web site address so that you can read about their practice. The cost associated with mailing information can be expensive. The cost of the printed material is expensive. Not to mention the cost of postage and the human resource staff that are required to handle the requests, shipping and handling. For this reason, some of the bariatric practices rely on the Internet to provide you with the most up to date information. Again, you will find that the Internet is an invaluable resource for gathering or retrieving data. If you do not have a personal computer, someone you know has a computer and they can help you with getting access to the Internet. Nearly every public library has public access to the Internet as well.

The Consultation

Once you choose a surgeon, your first step will be a consultation visit. Please prepare for this first meeting by reading all of their information. Highlight any part that you don't understand. Take a notebook and have your questions ready.

Before your consultation visit, I suggest that you get a copy of your medical records from the last five years from your PCP. If you have had any previous abdominal surgeries, I would get the medical notes for that as well. Take a list of your current medication and a list of all your allergies. Ask the office to send you their new patient questionnaire. Complete this form before your consultation visit. It is easier to fill out the form when you can spend some quiet time working on it. There are other things that you can take with you on this consultation visit. They are not necessary or required, but they are good things for the surgeon to include in your medical file, like the names and phone numbers of your supporters and a copy of a durable medical power of attorney.

Consultation Questions

(Some of these questions will be answered in the information packet.)

☑ Possible Questions
What testing do you require and when? (Blood test, EKG, gall stone ultrasound, upper GI, lung testing, chest x-rays, etc.)

☑	**Possible Questions**
	What should I do to prepare for the surgery?
	Do I have to do anything special the day before surgery like washing with special soap?
	Is there a special pre-op diet like clear liquids only?
	Do you require psychological testing? What type of mental health professional can do the psych eval? Does it have to be a doctoral level or masters level education? Do you offer suggestions?
	Any special instructions for smokers?
	Will sleep apnea interfere with surgery or recovery?
	What medications are given before and after surgery? What substitutes are there if I am allergic to them?
	Which gastric bypass surgery do you perform? Billroth II, RNY or DS?
	Will the surgery be done laproscopic or open?
	Do you use staples or sutures? Do you use special bands?
	Is the anesthesiologist experienced with large people?
	How much of the intestine is bypassed?
	Do you remove the gall bladder? Do you prescribe bile salts?
	What are the pre-op and post-op meds taken for?
	Will you do a liver biopsy if the liver looks bad?
	How long will I be in the recovery room?
	Will I get a patient controlled pain pump?
	How long will I have an IV?
	Will I have a nasal gastric tube? When will it come out?
	Will I have a catheter? When will it come out?
	Will I have any drainage tubes? When will they come out?
	How soon after surgery can I drink clear liquids?

☑ Possible Questions

For open incisions, are stomach binders provided at the hospital or should I bring my own?
Are there any surgical assistants? Who are they?
Will you visit with my family after the surgery to let them know how the surgery went? If there are privacy issues, can this meeting not take place?
Which hospitals do you perform surgery at?
When do I have to register at the hospital? Can I pre-register at the hospital?
When do I have to be at the hospital for surgery?
How do I find out my surgery time?
If I am coming from out of town, are there any hotel discounts?
How long is the hospital stay?
Are the gowns, wheel chairs and room chairs big enough for large people?
Will the staff be able to transfer large people?
Can I take any medication on my own at the hospital, like nasal spray or other over the counter relief aids?
How soon after surgery do most people have a bowel movement? Will I have to stay in the hospital until I have a BM?
Will I have a private room or will I have to share?
Can someone spend the night at the hospital with me?
How often should I walk after surgery?
What is the policy about nail polish and acrylic nails? Do they have to be removed?
What is the policy about jewelry during surgery?
Have you ever had a case where the surgery had started and you couldn't complete it? What are the chances of this?
What type of complications have you seen during surgery and post-op?
What are the possible surgical complications?

☑	**Possible Questions**
	How will my bowel patterns change?
	Will the bowel odor change?
	What short-term side effects should I expect?
	What long-term life changes should I expect?
	What vitamins do you recommend? Do you require vitamin and protein supplements?
	When are the incision staples removed?
	If traveling from out of town – what precautions should be taken after surgery?
	How much time should it take to recuperate?
	Do I have a limit on how much I can lift?
	How long before I can have sex?
	What will the scar look like?
	How much should I lose and how fast?
	How small will my stomach be? Will it stretch back out?
	What is dumping?
	What are the post-op diet instructions?
	Are there any foods I need to avoid?
	Do you have a support group? When are the meetings?
	Will I need to get monthly B-12 injections?
	How much water should I try to drink?
	What kind of exercise do you recommend after surgery and how soon can I start?
	Since I will not be able to take aspirin or anti-inflammatory drugs ever again what should I take instead? Do you have a list of what I can and cannot take?
	What about pregnancy after the surgery?
	When can I have children without risk to my unborn child or myself?
	Should I get a medic-alert bracelet?

☑ Possible Questions

	Is this surgery reversible? Have you ever done a reversal or a revision?
	How many operations have you performed?
	Can I have some patient referrals?
	How much is the total cost of the surgery?
	Have you had anyone with my insurance carrier and did they have any trouble getting approval for the surgery?
	Will you help during the appeal phase, if my insurance refuses the first request?
	If my insurance won't pay do you and the hospital have a self-pay rate?
	If I have to pay for the surgery or pay a co-pay, does this have to be paid before the surgery?
	Can I give blood since I will take iron the rest of my life?

Consultation Checklist

Use this checklist as a reminder for what you should take with you on your consultation visit.

☑ Item

	Medical records for the past five years
	Medical documentation from any past abdominal surgeries
	Name, address, phone number and fax number of your PCP
	The medical questionnaire already completed
	A list of your current medications including how long you have been on the medication, what you are taking the medication for, the dosage and how often you take the medication
	A list of your current diagnoses
	An allergy list
	Highlighted information from the information packet
	Your list of questions

☑	Item
	The completed copy of the qualifications checklist from Chapter Five
	A copy of your durable medical power of attorney form
	Names and contact information of your supporters
	A before picture
	A psych evaluation
	Recent lab test results
	The stomach diagram

Chapter Seven

"Well it all started with me feeling down AGAIN about my weight. I was at work and feeling depressed about being the biggest woman in the building. So I pulled up the Internet and went surfing. By the grace of GOD I found the clos.net website. I printed out everything I could find including pictures. I kept this information to myself for a couple of days and joined the email support list. When I started reading all the e-mails and made my first contact I was hooked. I printed out success stories and talked to a few more people before I approached my husband."

"We both needed to do this and I wanted to convince him that I had found the answer to our prayers. He was very skeptical at first but once he started reading the e-mails and talking to people himself he became as excited as I was. I was scheduled to go first, but I got laryngitis and I had to reschedule for another week. I broke down and cried. I was so ready."

"Rick went first. He was nervous but knew this was what he wanted to do. Eight months later Rick has lost 130 lbs. He has gone from a size 54 waist pant to a 34 waist pant. I have lost a total of 105 lbs. I went from a size 26 to a wonderful size 10 in just 8 months! Rick and I have never been happier. We have more energy, and food does not dominate our life. We live every moment to the fullest possible and thank God every day for the chance to live again."

Rick & Janet Armour
http://www.geocities.com/tricia_810/mgb/indiv/armours.html
Laparascopic Billroth II, May 2000

Dealing With Your Insurer...

My Soapbox

Most people have never taken the time to read their health insurance card let alone their health insurance policy. I was guilty of this myself. In this chapter, I am going to give you a step-by-step guide to follow. I wish I could guarantee that if you follow my steps to the "t" you will emerge successful. What I can tell you though, is that by following these steps, it puts you in a more powerful position to win your case with the insurance company. These are the very same steps that I took and I emerged the victor in my insurance battle... and it was a battle!

I will also tell you that many people unknowingly make some terrible mistakes early on when dealing with the insurance company by not getting any wise counsel first. And who can blame them? How are you to know that the insurance company may be your number one archenemy when you are expecting them to be your number one ally by paying for your surgery? I don't want to sound militant, but most insurance companies will count on you to be ignorant, timid and passive. They know that many people will not seek legal counsel and get tired of the fight and just give up. I can tell you that in my case, the insurance company appeared [to me] to do this deliberately and without shame. It reminds me of a joke I once heard. Three men go to heaven, the first was a doctor, the next was a social worker and the last fellow was a health insurance claims manager. St. Peter greets them at the gate and says, "Welcome Dr. Smith! You have done a wonderful job on earth helping the sick. You may enter!" The next man steps up and St. Peter says, "Welcome Mr. Jones! You have done a wonderful job on earth counseling the people in their hard times. You may enter!" The last man steps up and St. Peter says, "Welcome Mr. Clark! You have done a wonderful job on earth helping some people get medically necessary care. You may enter, but only for three days. After that you have to leave!"

Keep in mind that the predominant societal thought is that obesity is your fault and the treatment is to push yourself away from the table. The insurance industry is not immune to this philosophy. Pushing yourself away from the table costs the insurance company nothing. Paying for your surgery will cost them something, but so would the costs associated with you remaining morbidly obese. There are articles and studies that show that the insurance industry could save money [if you get the surgery] because of the costs associated with treating obesity-associated co-morbidities, like hypertension, gout, arthritis, type two diabetes, sleep apnea and cardiopulmonary problems. Still, the insurance industry has been reluctant to respect these reports and findings when they know that "fat people" die younger. In many cases they refuse to underwrite or insure morbidly obese people in order to avoid any health related costs of the "fat people." Maybe you've never experienced being denied health insurance coverage because you work for a big company or the government. But there are many people who are turned down for coverage everyday because of their weight. While large companies can afford policies that allow for "pre-existing conditions" like obesity, small companies don't have this same money or power. The insurance company does its best not to deal with "fat people" altogether.

Before I get into the steps you need to take, I want to spend some time educating you about the insurance industry. Even though the insurance industry is a "regulated" industry, the insurance company has a tremendous amount of latitude in making up their own rules. As outlined in Chapter Six, there are national guidelines established for the treatment of morbid obesity. The insurance company is under no jurisdiction to abide by these guidelines. They do not have to comply with, follow or adopt the guidelines established by the National Institute of Health or Milliman & Robertson. They can use them as a reference if they want, but that's it. The insurance company is seemingly well within its right to act as judge and jury when making up rules, writing in exclusions and wielding the power to give care to some and deny it to others. Many attorneys will tell you that the insurance company does have the right to set its own criteria, but they don't have the legal right to make up rules for the sole purpose of denying otherwise medically necessary care. They will tell you that if this is "proven" the case might be worth pursing and you could sue them. I am not an attorney. I have a healthy respect for the legal profession and I can tell you that the insurance company has deeper pockets than [most of] you. You can try to sue them, but that could wind up costing more money than it would cost to self-pay for your surgery. The average person doesn't have that kind of capital lying around. In addition, if the insurance company thinks you really have a case, they have the option to "shut you up" by paying for your claim, dragging the case out or hiring the best attorneys that money can buy. In addition, because they are able to lobby and give money politically, their connections can be very strong. The reason I mention this is not to discourage you from seeking legal counsel. In fact, I will often advise you to get an attorney. I just hear lots of people say "I'm going to sue the insurance company" and they need to know that suing them is not an easy task and it may cost them their life savings. If you find an attorney willing to fight and not charge you a dime, then sue them! The approach I will suggest is that you follow these steps methodically and purposefully and try to get your surgery covered. If you are able to do that, you can then help others to follow in your footsteps so that they too can get "approved" for surgery.

Develop Patience

Dealing with the insurance company can be a terribly stressful experience. I know this first hand. I strongly recommend that if you have to use insurance to get this surgery, you should pray for the best and prepare for the worst. Before you embark on your insurance journey, I want you to exercise patience, emotional control and stay calm. I want your attitude to be one of confidence. What I am about to share with you can be incredibly empowering. You have to know, believe and understand that the insurance company never has the power to determine whether you get surgery, they only have the power to pay for it. At all times, you must be empowered by the fact that the only thing standing between you and this life saving surgery is your determination and willingness to do "whatever it takes." If you have this attitude, I can guarantee that you will have this surgery with or without your current insurance carrier. I once learned that if the wall is to thick, then walk around it! If the wall is too long, then climb it! If the wall is too high, dig under it! If you really get in touch with this concept, nothing will keep you down, nothing at all! Your focus will be taken from a place of circumstance to a place of solutions. With confidence, you will do what needs to be done to get the job done. If you focus on the goal you will be amazed at how much peace you will have in the midst of an otherwise stressful journey.

Insurance Does Pay

The fact is, even though the insurance industry has a horrible reputation, they pay for gastric bypass surgery every single day. There are many good insurance policies that cover the surgical treatment of morbid obesity. This is not rare. If you are not on the Internet, I urge you to get access to the Internet. The Association of Morbidly Obesity Support at obesityhelp.com has a database of thousands of members who have shared their experience in dealing with your insurer. I also urge you to go to the bariatric surgeon's support group. There you will meet people who have gone through what you must go through. Finally, there's the office staff of the bariatric surgeon's practice. They will let you know early on which insurers are easy, difficult and impossible. Even if you find that you are dealing with an good insurer, I strongly urge you to follow these steps.

Finally... The Steps

Keep An Insurance Notebook

You want to start an insurance notebook so that all of your information is in one place. Find a notebook, binder or folder that has pockets and dividers. You want to keep your information organized as best as possible.

Never Ever Forget That This is Your Battle

Never depend on someone else to do your job. The insurance battle has no place for passivity. If something needs to be faxed, copied, mailed, checked, cross-referenced, called in, confirmed, verified, communicated, delivered or couriered, YOU DO IT! You must follow up on every little thing. You will find that you need access to a fax machine. If you don't have a fax machine, I suggest that you get one. Even if it means using Kinko's, your job or getting a free on-line fax number from efax.com. Remember at all times that nobody is going to benefit from your surgery more than you.

Read Your Policy

Get that insurance policy out, dust it off and read it. Your insurance policy may be lost; God knows it's not a book you read everyday. Even I had to hunt mine down. If you have lost your insurance book, you should be able to get a copy from the human resource benefits manager. You can also request another copy from the insurance company, but know that they update and add things to these books. What was originally in your book may have been taken out, revised or changed. Once you do find it, read it from cover to cover. Get a highlighter and pay special attention to the schedule of benefits, what's covered, what's not covered, out of network benefits, grievance procedures, complaints, appeals and exclusions. These are your key words. You are looking for anything in print that states if the policy covers obesity surgery, covers obesity treatment or excludes coverage for gastric bypass surgery or the treatment of obesity.

Three Findings

In reading your policy, you are going to find one of three things. Coverage for obesity and/or surgery is clearly stated, coverage for obesity and/or surgery is <u>not</u> clearly stated or coverage for obesity and/or surgery is definitely excluded. I encourage you to read over the content for all of the findings even if you know the answer about your own coverage.

Clearly Stated Coverage
And You Meet The Qualifications
If the coverage is clearly stated, then specific guidelines for obesity treatment should be listed. The guidelines are made very plain and you will be able to know if you meet the criteria and qualify for surgery or if you do not. If you qualify, you can start investigating which bariatric surgeons are available to you through your plan. If the bariatric surgeon of your choice is on the list, it seems like all systems are go.

First, call the insurance company as an information call. Get your insurance notebook out and write down the number you called, which buttons you had to push to get a human voice, who answered the phone and even who transfers the call if this is the case. Once you get someone who can help you, ask their name, extension number and direct dial number first before you launch into the conversation. Explain to them that you want this information just in case the call gets disconnected; you want to be able to call back without going through the same maze it took to get them on the phone. Don't tell them "I want gastric bypass surgery." Instead have them confirm what you have read about obesity treatment in your policy. Once they confirm that what you've read is accurate, tell them you think you may qualify for the surgery according to their guidelines. Ask this case manager or customer service representative what steps you need to take. Make sure to write down all of their responses including the date and time of your call. As you document their information, pay special attention to any instructions that may deviate from the coverage information in your book. If there are any discrepancies or seeming misinformation, ask them to explain the discrepancy. Tell them that this is not in your book and you can't find that in the manual anywhere. See if you can get them to put this in writing and fax it or mail it to you. Before ending your call, ask them if there is an alternate number to reach them in case their voice mailbox number is full. Try to get all of the possible contact numbers you can. Through my own experience, I have learned to expect that the insurance industry is good at giving mixed messages. You will never regret documenting the details.

Clearly Stated Coverage
And You Don't Meet The Qualifications
If you find that you don't meet the qualifications, it's your choice to try and continue to move forward. The worst thing that can happen is a denial letter. You may still qualify for the surgery based on the surgeon's patient criteria. If this is the case, you may want to read the next chapter on Financing Your Surgery.

Clearly Stated Coverage
And Your Surgeon (or Surgery) is Not On The List
If you find that your surgeon is not on the list, and many bariatric surgeons for good reasons will not be on the preferred provider list, you need to see if you have out of network benefits. It is particularly frustrating if you want a laparascopic minimally invasive approach and a laparascopic surgeon is not in the network. Likewise, it is equally as frustrating if you have your heart set on one particular surgery and your insurance company only covers the type you don't want. In these cases, you will have to go out of the network. Out of network benefits, when offered as a part of your plan, generally means you will have to pay for a larger portion of the bill than if you received the care in network. Some policies allow for the same coverage both in and out of network or if there is no one in network qualified to do the surgery. This will all depend on your policy. If this is your case, you will need to probe the case manager about your out of network benefits. There may be special rules and guidelines associated with out of network reimbursement. For example, the insurance company may choose to have you pay the up front expenses and then reimburse you when you go out of network. Be prepared. Don't make the mistake of trusting the case manager or customer service representative. If the rules for out of network care are not clearly stated, get it in writing. I repeat, get it in writing. The insurance companies are notorious for verbal agreements that aren't worth the paper they are written on. Did you catch that? Even with your notes and documentation, without something in writing, it's your word against the insurance company employee. Who do you think the insurance company will side with? You or their own employee? Especially when it comes to them reimbursing you. If they refuse to put the terms of coverage or reimbursement in writing, I would contact an attorney to make the request. The legal expenses associated with making a phone call or writing a letter is affordable. It's worth it if you can get that verbal agreement in writing. If you don't have out of network benefits and your heart is set and your mind is made up about a particular surgeon or surgery, read the next chapter on Financing Your Surgery.

The Dreaded Exclusion
When the Exclusion is Clearly Stated

An exclusion, as the word implies, is an agreement between you and the insurance company. The agreement was accepted before the policy took effect and it basically states that your insurance will not cover or exclude coverage of "these things." These things will be listed in the exclusions. Every insurance policy has exclusions. In fact, most of them have a longer list of what they exclude than things that they cover. Sometimes the exclusion is written clearly. If it is clearly written, it will state something like this – "Under no circumstances, whether medically necessary or not, we do not cover the treatment of obesity, morbid obesity and gastric bypass surgery." This type of exclusion is like a death nail in your weight loss surgery coffin. Many policies have this type of exclusion written in them and most morbidly obese people don't know it until the day they want weight loss surgery. If you are a human resource or benefits manager, don't agree to a policy that excludes weight loss surgery or the surgical treatment of morbid obesity. Morbid obesity is a disease and weight loss surgery is not experimental care. It is the only form of treatment that has positive long-term results. Nothing else has the outcome that gastric bypass surgery has for treating morbid obesity in the short-term or the long-term. For this reason, I beg the employers to block this exclusion. The health insurance quote will be higher without the exclusion, but not by much. It may be as little as two dollars a month more.

If your policy has an exclusion clause that is clearly stated, I do not recommend fighting it because it was an agreement made as a condition of the policy. The insurance company is not trying to harm you or even deny you medically necessary care. They may sympathize with you, agree that the care is medically necessary and understand your position. They may even cover any complications as a result of your surgery. But because the agreement is written so clearly, it is doubtful that they will cover your surgery.

Even with this exclusion, some people will try to get the surgery covered under their co-morbidities. If your obesity-associated diagnoses are bad enough, there is a chance that the surgery could be viewed as treatment for the other diagnosis. The hardest part about winning the insurance company over is that the treatment for each of the obesity related disorders is not gastric bypass surgery. The treatment protocol, whether it be lifestyle changes or medication will not be gastric bypass surgery. Instead, the insurance company can say that the reason you have the diagnosis may be because of your morbid obesity, but there is another way of treating it besides losing weight. They won't deny that losing weight would be good for treating the disease, but in many cases, they won't agree that the disease will be "cured" through the weight loss, much less the gastric bypass surgery.

If you try to get your surgery covered as a result of the co-morbidities, continue reading. The same steps required for approval whether the coverage for obesity was clearly stated, excluded or not clearly stated are the same. If the exclusion is upheld or you choose not to fight the insurance company, read the next chapter on Financing Your Surgery.

The Dreaded Exclusion
When the Exclusion is Vague or Conditional
My policy had an exclusion clause. It was not clearly stated. Instead it was vague and left an out for the treatment of obesity. My exclusion read, **"We exclude treatment or products for obesity, food addiction or weight reduction unless authorized by your physician through SummaCare's Health Services Management Program"**. Did you catch that end part? It says, "Unless authorized." All I cared about was getting the surgery authorized.

If your exclusion has an exception, conditional clause or is stated in vague terms, you may have a chance at getting your surgery covered. I was able to get my surgery covered with the exclusion written in my plan, but it was an awfully stressful experience. Even with daily prayer, meditation and confidence galore, this was no easy trek.

Exclusions need to be clear. If you try to get your surgery covered with the conditional exclusion continue reading. The same steps required for approval whether the coverage for obesity was clearly stated, excluded or not clearly stated are the same.

Whether the exclusion is clearly stated or conditional, I strongly urge you to call your case manager or customer service representative, just like you would if the coverage were clearly stated. Go back and read that section if you need to . What you want to do is engage the case manager in a conversation about what you've read in your policy book. Confirm if you are reading the exclusion correctly. Don't hesitate to ask the case manager if they know of anyone else who had the surgery covered with the same exclusion. I don't expect them to tell you if they had, so the worst they can do is lie.

When The Coverage is Not Clearly Stated
Whether the coverage is not clearly stated by an act of omission or through a vague or conditional exclusion, you now have to become Sherlock Holmes. Begin to investigate the hidden criteria that the insurance company guards like Fort Knox. This is what I had to do. My exclusion said that I needed to be "authorized" by my physician through the insurance company. My physician was a supporter, but I didn't know if I met the insurance company's patient criteria because I didn't know what the criteria was.

When the insurance company does not have any written qualification standards, or the wording is vague like "when medically necessary," this is a red flag. Do not assume that the insurance company will use the guidelines and standards from the National Institute of Health or Milliman & Robertson (you can find these standards in Chapter Five). You will have to be bold, confident, tenacious and straightforward when trying to get the guidelines from your insurance company. The insurance company is within their legal right to make up their own criteria. Your job is to get this criterion in writing BEFORE you submit your request for pre-authorization for surgery.

Let your request begin with a phone call to the case manager or to the customer service representative. Approach the subject by asking for the guidelines to be approved for gastric bypass surgery for the treatment of morbid obesity. Do not tell them you want this surgery let them assume it. Tell them you are investigating gastric bypass surgery. Tell them that while reading your policy book, you did not see any guidelines for gastric bypass surgery or the exclusion seemed have a conditional clause. When I called my insurance company, the customer service representative had a canned response. She told me that gastric bypass surgery for the treatment of morbid obesity was completely excluded. I explained that the policy stated that the treatment for obesity had to be authorized by the plan [according to the policy book I was reading]. Eventually the customer service representative admitted that she was given strict instructions that the insurance company would not authorize gastric bypass surgery for morbid obesity. There is a local bariatric surgeon in my area, so I called his office and spoke to his billing clerk. I asked her if my particular insurance company had ever paid for any of their patient's weight loss surgery. She told me nearly everyone had been denied. Even though many people had been denied, I knew what I read in my policy book and the exclusion was conditional. I wasn't going to give up that easy.

> *Never depend on someone else to do your job. The insurance battle has no place for passivity. If something needs to be faxed, copied, mailed, checked, cross-referenced, called in, confirmed, verified, communicated, delivered or couriered, YOU DO IT!*

I have come to expect that the insurance company guards the gastric bypass patient qualification information closely. I also believe that in many cases, the criteria are not in writing. They just seem to make them up as they go along on a case-by-case basis. This gives the insurance company a very unfair advantage because they have the upper hand in denying you based on essentially anything.

A phone call or a letter to get this information in writing is a good use of an attorney. It is worth the attorney's fee. Your other alternative is to contact the Department of Insurance (DOI) in your state. While it seems like the insurance industry has plenty of latitude and rights, it is a heavily regulated industry. Every state government has a DOI. Some states have great customer service and others are mediocre, it just depends on which state you live in. In the Appendix section of this book, I have listed the contact numbers for the DOI in your state. Keep in mind that the DOI will generally not fight for you. Your complaint to them is that your insurance company's policy is vague and they are unwilling to give you clarification in writing. Let your request to the DOI be very clear. You are not coming to them to get pre-authorized for surgery, because this is out of their hands. You want them to get those guidelines for you in writing since your policy is unclear. Between the attorney's request and the DOI, my guess is that you will have a very good chance of getting this information in writing. If the insurance company still does not cooperate in giving you these guidelines in writing, there is still one way left to find out their qualifications. It will be in a denial letter.

The Department of Insurance

Each state has a Department of Insurance, but they are not created equal. One role of the Department of Insurance is consumer protection. The laws regarding consumer protection vary from state to state. I didn't know anything about consumer protection laws until I started asking questions. I suggest that you contact your Department of Insurance and ask them if they have any pamphlets or brochures on consumer issues relating to health insurance. Some states, like Ohio, have laws that prevent an insurance company from being both judge and jury when it comes to determining medically necessary care. In Ohio, this law is called House Bill 4 and it was enacted in May 2000. This is how I won my case against my insurance company.

Submitting Your Request For Pre-Authorization

Each insurance company has their own way of making a pre-authorization or referral request. Some companies require the PCP to fax in a special form; some require the patient to initiate the call to the insurance company. Whatever the rules are regarding pre-authorization, follow them. But you need to make sure that before the authorization goes in, you have proof in hand that you meet all of the criteria. This proof should be part of the initial request for pre-authorization. In the Appendix section, you will find several sample letters that you can use as a guide when submitting your request for pre-authorization to the insurance company. Even though the "official" referral form may be one page, please submit a letter or other documentation along with the referral that shows that you meet the criteria. If your process for pre-authorization starts with a phone call, ask them if you can formally submit your request for pre-authorization in writing. Don't forget to document all of this and be detailed. Whenever you submit any documentation to the insurance company, try to get a receipt. If it is a fax, get a verbal confirmation the fax was received or a fax transmission report. If you send it in by mail, get very specific mailing information and use delivery confirmation so that you have signature evidence as a receipt. I have observed that some insurance companies are notorious for misplacing or losing documents. Whatever you send to the insurance company, be sure to make a copy for yourself with notes including who it was sent to and why it was sent. Document the date and the method of delivery. This is so very important.

Gather your list of criteria from your PCP, surgeon and the insurance company. If you want, you can use the guidelines established by other sources in addition to the PCP, surgeon and your insurance company. Next to each standard, guideline or criteria, write down how this can be proven and what evidence you have in writing. I strongly recommend that you do this exercise before you submit your first referral request or ask for pre-authorization.

Establishing Proof That You Meet The Criteria

In Chapter Five, I provided a checklist of patient criteria. Using this checklist, I am going to give you tips on how to establish written proof that you meet the criteria. Using your insurance notebook or binder, create a tab or section for each criteria. In each section, you are going to write out how you can prove that you meet the criteria. You will need a copy of your medical chart for this exercise. This exercise will be invaluable to you throughout your weight loss journey. Your notebook is personal, but it will also prove to be invaluable when you need to prove that you meet the criteria. My surgeon required a very similar task and I am grateful that he did.

Are you morbidly obese? Does your BMI exceed 40?
Morbid obesity is defined by the National Institute of Health as being 100 pounds overweight or having a body mass index (BMI) of 40 or more.

The nationally accepted height and weight tables that are nationally recognized are the Metropolitan Life and Health Insurance Height and Weight Tables. I have included this information in the Appendix. There are several web sites that offer a BMI calculator; I list three of the websites addresses in the Appendix. If you do not have immediate web access, the BMI can be calculated using this formula:

(The BMI guidelines use the metric system.)

You have to convert your height in inches to your height in meters.
Divide your height (in inches) by 39.36 to determine your height in meters
Example: 70 inches / 39.36 = 1.78 meters

You have to convert your weight in pounds to your weight in kilograms.
Divide your weight (in pounds) by 2.2 to determine your weight in kilograms
Example: 160 lbs / 2.2 = 72.73 kg

Multiply your height in meters by itself. This is called "squaring your height".
Example: 1.78 x 1.78 = 3.16

Divide your weight (in kilograms) by your squared height.
Example: 72.73 / 3.16 = 22.99

The BMI is 22.99 or you can round it off to the whole number, which is 23.

Proof of the fact that you are morbidly obese should be included in your medical chart. If you are heavier than the doctor's scale will weigh, there should be some evidence of this in the medical record. If you want to get an accurate weight, there are scales that do weigh in excess of 350 pounds. Though it may be horribly embarrassing to you, you can call around to some bariatric surgeons or hospitals and ask if they have a scale that measure in excess of the standard office scale, which weighs 350 pounds. Document your weight and BMI on the criteria checklist in Chapter Five.

Are you well informed?
A well-informed patient is one who is well-read. List all of the things you have read, researched and discussed as evidence that you are well informed. Ask your doctor to make a notation about this in the medical record.

Are you motivated? Do you strongly desire substantial weight loss?
Motivation is defined as action. Evidence of being motivated can be shown as a result of the documentation notebook that you started for your insurance journey. Again, ask your doctor to make a notation in the medical record. You can also make up a patient criteria checklist using the example in Chapter Five and have your physician sign it.

Have you accepted the operative risks?

The best way to evidence this is by writing down the operative risks. If you meet people in support groups that have had operative complications, you can write their name and contact information next to the complication and make some notes about their comments regarding their complications.

Are you able to participate in treatment? Are you able to participate in long-term follow-up?

This is a simple yes or no question, but I would like you to expound on why treatment and long-term follow up are important.

Do you think that the benefits for surgery outweigh the risks?

Make a list of the benefits you except to achieve as a result of having gastric bypass surgery.

Do you have any functional impairment associated with obesity? Has obesity impaired your quality of life? Do you have obesity-induced physical problems that interfere with your lifestyle?

Make a list of the physical and mental burdens that you endure as a result of your size. Go back to Chapter One and look at the list of physical and mental challenges.

Do you clearly and realistically understand how your life may change after the operation?

State how you think your life may change as a result of gastric bypass surgery. Later on, I'll explain the danger associated with false beliefs about losing weight.

Is your BMI over 35 with high-risk co-morbid conditions? Does obesity cause an incapacitating physical trauma as documented by the medical history records including x-ray findings and other diagnostic test results? Is there a significant respiratory insufficiency documented by respiratory function studies and blood gases? Is there significant circulatory insufficiency documented by objective measurements? Is there documentation that the management of primary diseases such as arteriosclerosis, diabetes and heart disease are complicated by the obesity?

Do you have hypertension, diabetes, sleep apnea, cardiovascular disease, arthritis, joint pain, back pain, musculoskeletal dysfunction, gastro-esophageal reflux disease (GERD), increased blood lipids, intracranial hypertension, infertility problems, urinary stress incontinence, lower extremity edema or swelling or poor circulation? If you have any of these co-morbid obesity-associated diseases, create a page for each one. List the date or the time when you can remember being diagnosed and by whom. State whether you are or have taken medication for this diagnosis. Include how you feel and how this diagnosis affects your life. Your medical record must include this information. Take the time to write down where information about the particular disease can be found in your medical record. You will probably need the help of a nurse or medical professional to get though the abbreviations, medical lingo and handwriting. If you have any lab or diagnostic tests that prove your diagnosis, include that information as well.

Have you been obese for at least five years?

This can be proven through the medical record. This is why you may need a medical record that dates back at least five years. If you do not have this, you can include documentation of the names of people who would testify that they have known you for five years and that you have been obese for five years. This is not as strong as the weight record in your medical chart, but it is better than nothing at all. You can also use records from any diet center you may have tried, like Weight Watchers or Jenny Craig.

Have you tried non-surgical methods of accomplishing weight reduction under a physician's supervision and have failed? Have you had any nutritional counseling? Have you had any exercise counseling?

Many people have never done a detailed diet history and many physicians don't think to include this information in the medical record. If they have then great! Highlight the information in your medical chart about past diets you have tried. You will also need to assemble a diet history of your own. In Chapter One, there is a list of diets and gimmicks, which for me was a walk down memory lane. You may not remember the exact dates that you tried the diet, but you want to try to remember the year and the results of the diet. Did you lose any weight? How long did you try the diet? Did anyone try the diet with you? If you lost weight, how long did you keep it off? Did you tell a doctor that you were on this diet? Was the diet medically supervised or something you tried on your own? Once you finish your diet history, I strongly urge you to submit it to your doctor and if you can, have it signed and put into your medical record.

Do you have a specific correctable cause for the obesity like an endocrine disorder?

This is a simple yes or no question. Some people are obese because of a specific disease of the endocrine system. If this is your case, gastric bypass surgery may not be indicated. When the endocrine disorder is under control, the obesity will tend to reverse itself. If you have an endocrine disorder, you would know it. The symptoms are complex and you would not be able to lead a "normal life". You would be under the care of an endocrinologist and it is likely that your thyroid tests would be abnormal. Diabetes is an endocrine disorder, but there is no correctable cause for diabetes.

Have you achieved full growth? Are you past adolescence?
This can be proven by your age. There are a few teenagers who have had gastric bypass surgery. The youngest that I am aware of is a 14 year old. Many surgeons will have you wait until you are out of the adolescent years to have surgical treatment. Your birth certificate is evidence of your age.

Are you at high risk for obesity-associated illnesses?
The answer is yes. Anybody morbidly obese is at a high risk of obesity-associated illness. Make a list of the obesity associated diseases and list the family members who have this disease. Further evidence of this is found in articles and reports. You can use these in your notebook and also use news clippings that you find that address information about obesity and obesity-associated illnesses.

Have you had a surgeon's preoperative medical consultation and approval?
Get a letter from your PCP that states that you meet the criteria and the recommendation of the surgery. I suggest that you create a criteria checklist and have your PCP and surgeon sign it. In the Appendix, you will find some letter examples. These letters are provided as a guideline for you. Some physician practices are busy and backed up with paperwork. If you give them a sample letter that they can sign or that they can follow as a guide, it will expedite your process. Remember, this is your journey and your responsibility. Telling the doctor you need a letter is not good enough.

Have you had preoperative psychiatric consultation and approval? Have you had any psychological counseling?
The psychiatrist or psychologist who does your psych evaluation will write a letter recommending you for the surgery. There's a sample letter in the Appendix section.

Have you participated in any support group discussions?
List the support groups that you have attended whether it is in person or on-line. The groups don't have to be formal. Perhaps you met with some people who had gastric bypass surgery over dinner. This is a support group. You can also list support groups that you've attended in the past

like Overeaters Anonymous, Weight Watchers or a support group at your church. The support group doesn't have to be for obesity only. Support is support. Also include a list of your "supporters" in this section of your notebook as well.

Waiting On The Determination

Now that you have your notebook with evidence that you meet the criteria and the formal request for pre-authorization is in the hands of the insurance company, you have to wait on their determination. The insurance company has the right to have time to make a determination. It can take them up to 30 or 45 days. Waiting on their decision may be the most uncomfortable part of the entire process. During this process, it is all right to call and check on the request status. There's a difference between checking on the status and stalking. Your checking on the claim may not help the time frame in which they make the decision, but it does show them your determination and motivation.

The Determination

The determination will be one of three things. Approved, approved with conditions or denied. You may learn about your determination by phone or my mail. Depending on the news, your emotions can range from jubilant all the way down to despair. Denials are heartbreaking, disappointing, frustrating and stressful. This combination can push some people over the edge. I suggest that you have good support around you. I received three consecutive denial letters before that glorious day when I finally got approved.

Approved
I don't want to sound like a party pooper. When you get the notification that you have been approved, it is a time for celebration. But the question of cost still remains. Depending on your status of in network or out of network, complete coverage or partial coverage, an approval still has to be followed up with some more detail. It is important to get your approval in writing. Let me tell you a little story about my day of surgery. I wasn't the first one on the list for surgery that day, but I was bumped up to the first spot because the lady before me didn't have the approval letter and codes written, as the hospital needed it written. Her surgery was delayed on technicalities. Also keep in mind that pre-authorizations are usually dated. They are only good until a certain date. Many bariatric surgeons are booked solid, some have a waiting period of three months or more! If this is the case, make sure you get an extension on the date of your pre-authorization. So that you won't have any surprises, you need to clearly know and understand what is going to be covered and what is

going to be your responsibility. What are your deductibles, co-pays, percentages and maximum out of pocket expenses. The fees associated with surgery are going to be for the surgeon, the hospital and the anesthesia group. You should request a letter from the insurance company addressing at least these three components and be sure to have them include the procedure code. Every surgery has an CPT and ICD-9 procedure code. You can get this by calling your surgeons office. These procedure codes are important to the surgeon, anesthesia group and the hospital. As a precaution, you want to make sure that coverage is also extended to any complications as well.

Approved With Conditions (Strings Attached)

Some insurance companies give conditional approvals and some even set forth guidelines that will only allow surgery after you have had six months of nutritional counseling or some other requirement. These can be terribly frustrating. Some insurance companies may send an approval pending additional psychiatric or psychological counseling. Again, the longer the delay of surgery, the more frustrating the process. You might be approved for the gastric bypass surgery, but not with the surgeon of your choice. Likewise you may be approved for one procedure, but not the surgery of your choice. Either way, an approval with strings is often better than a denial. If you are approved, with strings, and the conditions are successfully met, you want to follow the same advice offered above under "Approved". Remember to document everything and get it all in writing. If you don't want to meet their conditions or you disagree with them, you can appeal. Continue reading, appeal information is included under "Denied".

Denied (Based On Exclusions)

A denial based on exclusions can be appealed. Every insurance company has an appeal process and a grievance and complaint process. The rules regarding appeal rights are in your policy book. You are allowed a limited number of appeals, usually two or three, but once all of the appeals are exhausted, the fight is usually over. You can start the process over again or you can seek legal counsel. If the policy exclusion was well stated, it will be hard to overturn. If it was vaguely stated, there may be room to win. I was first denied based on the exclusion, but when I appealed I was able to win the fact that the exclusion was vaguely written. Denials based on exclusions do not take medical necessity into account, therefore it is unlikely that any information about whether the surgery is medically necessary or not will be in the denial letter. Your appeal should focus on the fact that the exclusion is not clear and you believe you are not excluded. It may be helpful to get an attorney to draft an appeal letter. I have included a sample letter in the Appendix.

Denied (Based On Medical Necessity)

If you have done everything in your power to show the insurance company that you meet the criteria for surgery, and you know that you have left no stone unturned, then this denial letter from the insurance company will be of particular importance to you. The reason is most insurance companies will let you know that you are being denied because you don't meet some named criteria. If the insurance company was unwilling to share their full list of criteria with you after a request from the Department of Insurance and after a request from an attorney, it will be interesting to see what they put in this denial letter. If you know that you do not meet this named criteria in the letter, you may choose to give up your fight. If you do meet the criteria in the denial letter, you can seek more evidence that you meet these criteria and resubmit the request in the form of an appeal. A denial letter should include information on how appeal. As with the first request for pre-authorization, you will have to wait out the determination processes. In some cases, a carefully planned appeal packet will result in a victory and approval. I would enlist the help of an attorney to help you write the appeal letter and review your appeal packet. It is important to know that the insurance company's rationale for your denial should be included in the appeal letter. If the rationale is unclear to you, you can ask for further clarification in writing. Remember to document everything. If your initial request was limited to a referral letter and not your medical chart, submit your appeal request with a copy of your chart as well as the proof of evidence from the notebook you worked on for this weight loss surgery journey. Make sure that you submit it in a well-organized and professional fashion. Include a personal letter (see an example in the Appendix) and photographs as well as support letters from your supporters. The appeal process can be grueling. Remain calm, submit your packet and wait for the determination.

At some point in the denial and appeal process, you may be given the opportunity to appeal your case in person. One of the greatest fears that people have is public speaking. An in-person appeal will involve you speaking to a group of people from the insurance company about your case. If you have the opportunity to get an in-person appeal, I suggest that you go for it. The insurance company representatives may want to ask you questions during the in-person appeal, but they will also allow you to give them a speech about your appeal. I suggest that you gather your notebook and all of your evidence files that prove that you are a good candidate for weight loss surgery. Outline what you want to say using bullet points. Explain everything in your notebook from start to finish. Start with your history of obesity and the obesity-associated burdens you face on a daily basis. Move into an explanation of why you know you are a good candidate for the surgery and close by showing them that whatever reasons they offered as a reason to deny you this life-saving surgery are invalid. You are allowed to take a supporter with you to the in-person appeal. Your attorney might be a good choice. Practice your speech and be well prepared. Although you may be nervous about public speaking and you may feel embarrassment about sharing your life struggle about your obesity, the in-person appeal may be the step that is needed for approval. Be calm, be prepared, be thorough and be confident. This is your chance to look in the face of those who have the authority to pay for your surgery and you want to let them know that you have a life worth living and you don't want it cut short by carrying around an extra 100 pounds or more.

Don't ever stop appealing. Exhaust every appeal right and see if the state department of insurance has additional appeal rights beyond that of the insurance company. You are in a battle for your life. Once you have done everything you can and denial is still the outcome, move on to the next chapter, Financing Your Surgery.

Last Minute Thoughts

I've seen some approval processes take as little a two days and as much as two years. Patience is a must if you are in the latter group. Keep in mind that people are waiting for approval and their experience is much worse than yours. If you get a quick approval, remember to pray for those still waiting and always offer words of support and encouragement. Don't misunderstand if someone can't immediately rejoice with your quick approval, especially if they've been denied or are in the process of waiting. It's not that they aren't happy for you. They want that same blessing and it's not happening the same for them. If you are in a long approval process or if you have been denied, try to rejoice with the others even though you may be sad. If rejoicing is too much, at least offer some words of encouragement and share what you are going through.

Every "i" Dotted, Every "t" Crossed

Once you have your pre-authorization in hand, written as you need it with the appropriate dates, codes and benefit amounts outlined, you can start your journey. Perhaps you've already had your consultation or maybe you are waiting until you have proper authorization for your consultation visit. Either way, your next step is surgery.

The Insurance Checklist

☑	Insurance Checklist
	Develop patience
	Start an insurance notebook and document everything in it
	Never forget that this is your battle
	Read your policy book
	Determine if coverage is available to you
	Confirm the findings with the insurance company
	Establish proof that you meet the criteria
	Submit your request for pre-authorization
	Pray for approval
	Prepare for denial and the appeal process

Chapter Eight

"I have spent my whole life battling weight and am tired of being tired! I am active for a person of my size, but not active enough to chase my kids around the playground! I feel like I am always missing out and want to get back to the days when it took a lot to tire me out! I don't want my weight to be the focus of my every thought anymore. I have hoped for years to find a "cure" to my problem and finally I feel there is hope!"

Kjay Hellings
Laparoscopic DS, 10/6/2000

Financing Your Surgery

A friend once told me that she was so poor she couldn't even pay attention.

For many Americans, the thought of self-paying for gastric bypass surgery seems completely out of reach. But my on-line research indicates that upwards of 25% of all gastric bypass surgeries are done on a self-pay basis. The cost of self-paying for gastric bypass surgery will range from $13,200 to $35,000 (or more). If you are reading this and you are like my friend (who was too broke to pay attention), I know that raising this amount of capital may seem impossible. And if you factor in your credit status, existing debt and the overwhelming feelings of doubt about raising this amount of money, it does seem insurmountable.

If you do have to self-pay, there are tax incentives for you. Check with your tax specialist to learn how you can use the cost of surgery as a substantial deduction!

Best Gastric Bypass Deals For The Self-Payers

I did some investigative research and found the best surgeons offering the best self-pay rates on gastric bypass surgery. I've listed every type of bypass surgery and the best rate I could find. All of the surgeons listed have excellent track records. The prices may be low, but their service is top notch. The reason some surgeons can offer discount self-pay prices are because they've worked on your behalf to work with the hospitals or surgery centers to negotiate the best rate possible.

Keep in mind that these are the rates as of the printing of this book. You will have to call their office to see if these rates still apply. None of the surgeons listed are bound by the rates printed in this book.

Open Roux-en-Y Gastric Bypass
Dr. Paul M Selinkoff & Dr. John Pilcher
San Antonio, Texas
(210) 614-3370
$13,200
Web Site: http://www.sabariatric.com

Laparascopic Billroth II (Mini-Bypass)
The Center For Laparascopic Obesity Surgery
Dr. Robert Rutledge
Durham, North Carolina
(919) 479-1741
$14,000
Web Site: http://www.clos.net

Laparascopic Roux-en-Y Gastric Bypass
Laparascopic Weight Loss Surgery Center
Dr. Douglas Zinni
Las Vegas, Nevada
(702) 895-9452 or Toll Free (866) 895-9452
$17,000
Email: trish_l@lvcm.com

Open Duodenal Switch
Dr. John P. Maguire
Kettering, Ohio
(937) 534-0339 or Toll Free (888) 532-THIN
$23,000.00
Web Site: http://www.newlifesurgery.com

Laparascopic Duodenal Switch
Dr. Michel Gagner, Dr. Daniel M. Herron
Dr. W. Barry Inabnet III & Dr. Alfons Pomp
New York, New York
(212) 241-3699
$23,960.00
Web Site: http://www.surgicallyslim.com

Also keep in mind that complications may cost more. You will have to check with each practice to learn more about their costs and services.

How Am I Going To Pay For This Surgery?

Asking for money is humbling. It sets you up for disappointment if the person you are asking is unwilling to help. If you ask to borrow money, expect a no and rejoice in a yes. Pray for the best and prepare for the worst. Don't hold a grudge against those who cannot or will not help.

Change Jobs

If you can, move to a company with better health coverage. As you research which insurers cover gastric bypass surgery, start looking for a job that offers that coverage. In some cases, you may not have to change jobs; you may want to get a second job. Many part-time jobs have health insurance coverage but you have to pay the full monthly premium. This is a considerable amount less than paying for the entire cost of the surgery.

Talk To The Human Resource Manager

Some employers are unaware that they signed a policy with a gastric bypass exclusion. Ask the benefits manager to look into changing the policy. The insurance company will charge a higher premium with less exclusions, but it may only be a couple of extra dollars per employee per month.

Using Insurance Coverage For Gall Bladder Surgery Or Other Associated Fees

If your surgeon is one that removes the gall bladder, you may be able to get the "gall bladder surgery" covered and pay the surgeon the fees associated with the gastric bypass. The surgeon's fee can start as low as $3,500. This is far less than paying for the entire cost of the surgery.

There are other costs that may be covered by your insurance, like the cost of the psych evaluation or other lab tests. Just because your insurance has denied or excluded the gastric bypass does not mean that they can deny the complications associated with the surgery. Check with your insurer to learn what associated fees are covered.

Home Equity Loans

The advantage of a home equity loan is that the interest is tax deductible. In addition, the loan can be amortized over a longer period of time making your payments small.

Borrow From Family, Friends & Associates

If you borrow from this group, remember to get it in writing! These are the same people you will visit every holiday.

Ask Your Church

Some churches may have benevolent funds available to help with medical expenses for their members. Don't quit your church if they don't have money to help you.

Borrow Against Your Retirement

Check with your financial planner to see what borrowing options are available to you. In some cases, you can borrow interest and penalty free against your own retirement money.

Teaching Hospitals, New Surgeons

Surgeons who are already doctors (not medical students) are in training from existing gastric bypass surgeons. They may offer substantial discounts if you are willing to be a surgical patient. Keep in mind that these are already qualified surgeons. They are NOT students. Contact the bariatric surgeon and ask if they have any "surgeon students" in training.

Sell Something

Is there anything you own that you could sell? Luxury items that you don't use are a good place to start. Got a camper or boat you don't use? You can sell smaller items on eBay.

Use Credit Cards

I hate the high interest rate associated with credit card debt. But if I thought my life depended on this surgery, I'd accept the debt and work hard to pay it off as soon as possible. Perhaps you might only need to use the credit card for a portion of the surgery and not the whole thing.

Use Your Tax Refund

If you are getting a tax refund, use this money towards your surgery expenses.

Fundraisers

You can raise some of your money through fundraisers. If you have enough people who can help you, you can raise a couple thousand dollars.

Get Sponsors (Sponsor-a-Pound Campaign)

This is probably the most creative idea. You can divide the amount of the surgery by the number of pounds you need to lose. Let's say you have 150 pounds to lose and you need $12,000 for your surgery. That's $80 a pound. You can have people "sponsor-a-pound" to help you with your surgery. Their gift won't be tax deductible, but they can help you all the same. Create a one-page letter explaining your need for surgery and ask people, companies and charities to "sponsor-a-pound."

A Light At The End Of A Dark Tunnel

There is just one rainbow at the end of the self-pay storm. Our current tax law allows for a significant write-off or deduction for medical expenses when the medically related expenses are greater than 7.5% of your income. Check with your tax accountant or tax preparer to learn more about this tax law.

A Word About Being Overwhelmed

I know you may be overwhelmed with the thought of self-paying. If none of these suggestions work for you, and you firmly believe that this surgery is for you, you will find a way.

Chapter Nine

"Dieting gave me temporary success. I did lose some of the extra pounds, but shortly afterwards , the weight I lost came back and more! As soon as I relaxed the diet ritual – Wham! The weight loss became, weight gain. Then I began to see myself as a failure. This caused me to start eating to console myself. What a vicious cycle, I was getting fatter so I would get depressed."

"For several years I was able to lose some weight. But mostly, I was just glad that I was not gaining weight. But then it all started to fall apart – I started to gain weight and I just could not stop it. I starved, I suffered and I gained. I tried tailored clothes, I tried baggy clothes, I tried everything and I failed. I had to give up the diet business."

"This operation was the turning point in my life."

Daryl Davidson
http://members.tripod.com/Daryl_D/page01m.html
Open RNY, 11/1998

After The Consultation

Dealing With The Old You And Preparing For The New You

In Chapter Six, Selecting Your Surgeon, I explained the consultation visit with the surgeon. The time between the decision to have surgery (or your consultation) and your surgery date is not a time to kick up your heels and relax; it's the perfect time to begin to deal with the old you while preparing for the new you. As you move closer to the day of surgery, your greatest wish and prayer for a normal size body are well within your reach. The day you have fantasized about is going to become a reality and your life is going to change.

Bariatric Beliefs

I want you to have a wonderful weight loss surgery experience. I want you to have victory over the physical and mental burdens associated with being morbidly obese. If you go back to Chapter One, many physical and mental burdens are listed.

Normal size people take the benefits of living life in a normal size body for granted everyday. They don't think twice about zipping through turnstiles or shopping in a normal size store. Day in and day out they just go about their business without giving a second thought about how difficult life can be for us morbidly obese folks. I understand how they can do this because the majority of the time I don't give a second thought about how difficult my life would be if I were blind or deaf. It's not that I am insensitive about the needs of someone else, but I take sight and hearing for granted. For the readers who have good vision and hearing, take some time to thank God for these gifts, because they are priceless and precious gifts that you use every single day. [Myself included.]

My point however, is that relatively soon after your surgery; you will begin to take advantage of the benefits of living in a normal size body. It's easy to intoxicate yourself on the good feelings and thoughts of being a normal size. It's also easy to commingle the benefits of life in a normal size body with the false beliefs about being a normal size person. I call these false beliefs the fantasy traps.

The Fantasy Traps

There are many fantasy traps. They are like snares that will snag your joy about your transforming physical frame. I'm going to touch on just a few of these fantasy traps. I want you to make a list of your expectations about life after surgery. I hope to give you something to think about to help you discern whether your expectation is a real benefit of life in a normal size body or if it is a fantasy trap.

Fantasy Trap Number One
"I'm No Longer Going To Be Single"

I don't know if you are physically beautiful or not, but many fat women hear "You have such a pretty face." I have come to hate this halfhearted compliment. What is implied is that your face is pleasant to look at, but the rest of your body is not. To be honest with you, I agreed with them. I was disgusted with my size. I was never satisfied with my body and I suspect that I'll never have the type of body I really want. I think this is a human condition. We are rarely if ever fully satisfied with our own body. Even the celebrities we label as "perfect" candidly share that they are dissatisfied with one thing or another.

It is very easy to believe that as you lose weight, more people will be attracted to you. Those same people who tell you that you have such a pretty face are quick to tell you that the "men" will come out of the woodwork. They tell you that you'll have to beat them off like flies. And it's not just other people telling you this, we tell ourselves this. Sometimes we are expecting that people who don't find us attractive before surgery will all of a sudden find us attractive.

The rest of the fantasy goes something like this. Your admirers will be smitten by your new look, you'll play hard to get, they'll pursue you heavily, you'll eventually give in to their charms, the two of you will get married (being rescued from your life of singleness) and you'll live happily every after.

Yes, I'm being a little sarcastic, but only to make a point. Many people have blamed their single status on their size. While it is true that people are visual and obesity is often viewed as ugly, this is NOT the cause of your singleness. If you don't believe me, take a look around you and look at all of the normal sized single people. There are many of them. There are millions of dateless and mateless normal size people. If you were able to poll them, none of them would be able to use the excuse of morbid obesity for their singleness.

I want to point out that being normal sized will increase the number of people who will find you attractive, but that will not translate into meeting, (much less marrying) Mrs. Wonderful or Mr. Right. In fact, one of the things you will have to deal with when you lose weight is learning how to discern if an admirer is for real or not. In addition, being normal sized will increase your pool of Mr. & Miss Wrong.

Poor relationship skills are the cause of poor relationships. I know plenty of obese people. Some have good marriages and others are in bad marriages. If you want a good marriage, you need to start working on the skills that make a relationship work. I can guarantee you that there is nothing done in the surgery or the operating room that will help you become more loving, kind, patient or forgiving. These are the skills you need to cultivate to be a good spouse.

Obese, especially morbidly obese people experience a lot of rejection. Normal size people are not immune to rejection. You will still have to deal with rejection for the rest of your life. Don't fall into the fantasy trap that tells you that your admirers won't reject you because of your new physical frame. People can and will reject you regardless of your size.

Fantasy Trap Number Two
"My Marriage Will Be Better, My Spouse Will Love Me More"

If bariatric surgery could do this, every husband and wife regardless of their starting weight would gladly get on the operating table. This fantasy trap is a close cousin to fantasy trap number one. Your surgery transforms only your physical frame. It cannot and will not transform the mental or emotional frame of the people around you, especially your spouse.

Your spouse may respond positively to your weight loss or they may respond negatively. They may have fallen into some fantasy trap of their own. They may be thinking that you will become more sensual and sexual. You may think you'll become more sexual. But what if you don't? The issue is not how sensual you will become; it's how sensual you are now. If your sex life before surgery was boring, dull and not good, weight loss surgery will not improve it. But if your sex life is already good before surgery, it could get better because it's easier to move a normal size body. If you are ashamed to undress before your spouse because you are obese, what makes you think you will be more comfortable showing off sagging skin? The issue here is about your own shame, issues about the rejection from your spouse and a marriage that may lack emotional and sexual intimacy. The bariatric surgeon can't help these things.

Some spouses have a hard time dealing with the weight loss. They may be happy for you in some ways, but they may feel more vulnerable since there may be more admirers. They may also become intimidated as you gain confidence in your transformed body.

Since I'm here, I may as well add that you may find yourself more susceptible to affairs as the attention comes your way. Like the single person, you will have to find yourself exercising discipline, wisdom and self-control to guard against the infectious and intoxicating good feelings that come from newfound admirers.

Fantasy Trap Number Three
"I Can Eat Anything I Want"

I hate to burst your bubble, but you have to exercise self-control over your eating even after this surgery. Just as normal size people cannot eat a diet of high fat, high cholesterol and high sugar foods, neither can or should you. There are serious consequences to not following your dietary restrictions and guidelines.

It is true that your stomach is smaller than before and you physically cannot eat as much as before. You can choose to fill that new small stomach with unhealthy fats and carbs or healthy food choices. Keep in mind that surgery is a tool. A hammer by itself cannot build a house. Somebody has got to use the tool to make the tool effective. You have to use this tool to make weight loss effective.

Like you, before surgery, I tried diet after diet and I could lose weight, but I couldn't keep it off. To lose weight, I had to follow dietary restrictions. The beauty of weight loss surgery is that it is a really good tool to help you lose weight. It is virtually the only tool that will help you keep the weight off. The beauty of a hammer is that it is shaped and designed perfectly to do the job of pounding a nail. The diets and gimmicks that I used in the past to try to lose weight and keep it off was the wrong tool. It was like trying to use a pair of pliers to drive a nail into a piece of wood. Pliers are a good tool, but they are horrible at driving nails! Those other diets and gimmicks were like a pair of pliers to me when what I needed all along was a hammer.

You have to follow your nutritional guidelines. Each surgeon has their own recommendation and I will offer my two cents in Chapter Eleven, Post Op Living. What I want you to know is that you can eat anything (as long as you can tolerate it), but not everything is good for you. You won't need super human will power, but you will have to exercise good judgment and self-control in your food choices.

Fantasy Trap Number Four
"I'll Be Happy"

Happiness is terribly fleeting. The wind cannot be captured in your hand, and like the wind you cannot capture happiness in your life. What you can strive for instead of happiness is peace, joy and contentment. These three things are not like the wind. They can be captured because peace, joy and contentment are an attitude and a mindset that can be attained as a result of your good life choices. If you don't invite havoc into your life, you will have a better chance at attaining peace, joy and contentment.

You will be happy that you are losing weight, but those happy feelings won't last. Like a cool breeze or a gentle wind, they'll flow in and out of your life as you are losing weight. I urge you to develop a life that cultivates peace, joy and contentment. You can have this attitude regardless of your body size. Bariatric surgery will never be able to give you peace, joy and contentment, much less sustained happiness.

Wellness and becoming well will give you good feelings about yourself, but you should be warned that many people find themselves depressed after surgery. Like postpartum depression, it is hard to believe that after an event so great you can find yourself overwhelmingly sad. There are many reasons for this depression. The emotional upheaval of the event can cause depression. The grieving of your old body can be depressing. Fat has been an adjective to describe some of you since childhood and now that adjective is going to be stripped away. You will have to redefine and adjust to the new you. For many people, its overwhelming and depression can set in.

Estrogen is stored in the fat cells. This amount of estrogen can cause mood swings and depression. Some women need hormone therapy to control the ravages of free flowing estrogen. As you begin to lose weight fast, estrogen becomes free flowing. You can be "Fertile Myrtle" during this time.

When false expectations (the fantasy traps) go unmet or unfulfilled, depression can be the result. For all of these reasons and more, depression can be a reality and a part of your post-op experience. I strongly suggest that you find an accountability person to monitor your mood. This person can let you know if you seem to be slipping into some depressive moods. You will need support, but you may also need a counselor. Depression can be treated with psychotherapy, medication therapy or a combination. I do recommend though that before you begin taking antidepressants, check with your gynecologist to see if part of your depression is caused by a high level of free-flowing estrogen. The medication of choice might be hormone therapy and not antidepressants. The hormone imbalance will not last forever, it will resolve itself as the weight loss stabilizes.

Fantasy Trap Number Five
"I'm Going To Be Outgoing"

Our personality make-up is as genetic as our eye color. You are who you are. If you are an extrovert, you are because God made you that way and you'll be extroverted if you are fat, skinny or anywhere in between.

Obesity, especially morbid obesity, can cause lots of guilt, shame and embarrassment. As a result, you'll be less likely to participate in some physical activities because your size makes it prohibitive. Likewise, there are times you may decide to become a hermit during your own pity party moments. This behavior is NOT a result of an extrovert turned introvert.

Extroverts cannot help themselves from being outgoing. They are compelled to be outgoing. Maybe they can't do all the physical things and maybe they have a pity party every now and then, but extroverts are known for their presence. They are not shy, bashful or timid. They want their presence known. When I think of obese extroverts, I think of Carnie Wilson and Oprah Winfrey. Carnie and Oprah may not have liked their obesity, but it didn't stop them from being the extroverts that they are.

Bariatric surgery will not change your core personality traits. The introvert may become a little less introverted. And the extrovert will probably become a little bit more extroverted. But the extrovert and the introvert will not swap places. There are real physical burdens and challenges for the morbidly obese and once the weight is off, the physical challenges or barriers are no longer a hindrance to you. Just because you can participate, doesn't mean you will participate in any physical activity or embark on a lifelong dream.

One Last Word About The Fantasy Traps

I want you to have an awesome weight loss journey. I want this to be one of the most significant and special life events you experience. If you keep the expectations realistic and avoid the pitfalls of the fantasy traps, I am certain that life after surgery will be filled with rewards, pleasant surprises and good things. The road to morbid obesity was paved with many horrible emotions and memories. The road to a normal size body will be paved with many new victories, both big and small, which will give way to very pleasing new memories.

A Memory In The Making...

Life will change relatively fast. After surgery, the excess weight will come off in the first two years. Most people will be normal sized within the first year. Because this physical transformation happens so quickly, you can forget to document and record the journey until it's too late.

Before surgery, begin to make a memory through your own documentary. You'll never regret having a record of where you came from and seeing how far you've come. This documentary will also serve as a treasured keepsake to help you encourage others who you meet that struggle with morbid obesity.

Take Pre-Op Pictures

Take pre-op pictures with a full front, side and back view. Taking photos is awfully painful for many morbidly obese people, but this is one time when you don't want to run from the camera. Wear clothing that will contrast with the background. Pay close attention to what you decide to wear in these official pre-op photos because you want to save this outfit. As you share your story and show the before pictures, show the outfit that you wore in the pre-op photo. This outfit will become a part of your documentary out of obesity. From time to time, try the outfit on just to see how far you've come. When you reach your goal weight, take another post-op set of pictures wearing this same outfit in your new normal size body. The clothes will be hanging off of you and you'll probably have to hold up the pants. No words can describe the feelings of accomplishment and victory you feel as you stand in clothes that used to fill out your morbidly obese frame.

If you have photos that show when your obesity started, include them in your personal weight loss surgery photo album. My personal album starts with my baby picture. Under the baby picture I wrote, "I was born weighing six pounds, seven ounces and I've been trying to get back there ever since". The rest of my photo album includes photos from my youth, adolescence and adulthood right up until the day I had surgery.

As you start losing weight, take photos every month or every other month. Pose with the same front, side and back view and hold a sign that shows your weight and the date. Take these photos until you reach your goal weight. You can also choose to make a weight loss surgery video documentary.

Start A Journal

You've already started the insurance notebook (if you followed my advice). You can use this notebook or start another journal to chronicle your weight loss journey. You don't have to write a book, but it's important to record your thoughts, emotions and victories along the way. I've titled my journal "Along The Weigh - My Thoughts & Reflections Through Weight Loss Surgery". One of my early victories was fitting into a particular ugly green office chair with arms. This victory journal will become very encouraging as you reach plateaus in your weight loss.

Take Pre-Op Measurements

One friend told me that when you hit weight loss plateaus, your body is losing inches. I don't know if this is true, but it is encouraging to measure parts of your body and pull the tape measure tighter every couple of months. Before surgery, measure your neck, arms, wrists, bust line or chest, abdominal girth at the naval, hips at the widest point, thighs, knees, calves and ankles. Even your shoe size will decrease as you lose weight!

Start A Web Site At Obesityhelp.com

Eric Klein has done an extraordinary job creating and maintaining the on line Association for Morbid Obesity Support. You may not have a computer or you may be computer illiterate, but his web site is so well put together that sharing your story is as easy as typing or using a mouse. If you can't type or use a mouse, someone you know does and they can help you set up your free web page in under an hour. The reason I am able to share my story is because others had the courage to share their story. Your story will encourage untold millions. Talk about impact and making a difference!

Participate In Ongoing Support

Whether on-line or in person get involved in a support group before surgery and continue to participate in the support group after your surgery. There's always someone to encourage. Share your photo album and tell your personal story about how you overcame obesity.

Pre-Surgery Preparation & Recommendations

Align Support For Home & Family

Your recovery time and your postoperative hospital stay will depend on your age and health, but also whether your surgery is done open or laproscopically and if there are any complications. In most cases, you can return home within one or two days after a laparascopic surgery and four to five days after an open surgery. The open surgery patient will have more tissues that need to heal than the laparascopic patient, but both patients did have major surgery and a recuperative period should be recognized and respected. Take off adequate time whether it is a week or four weeks. Align support systems before surgery for help with childcare, housekeeping, chores and other day-to-day responsibilities. Don't overdo it. Keep your expectations realistic and listen to your body. Do what you can and get plenty of rest. Keep the names and phone numbers of your helpers, the doctor, surgeon and hospital nearby. Also, find a pharmacy or store that delivers. Call on help when you need it.

Clean That House Before Surgery

Don't come home to a torn up house. Do the laundry, cleaning and cooking before surgery. Prepare food in advance for the family and freeze it to make it easy on you after surgery. Stock up on household goods like soap, toilet paper, fabric softener and paper towels. You might not want to go out to the store and carry this stuff back in the house upon returning home after surgery.

Buy Your Food

For the first three weeks post-op, you will be on a clear liquid and soft diet. Don't bother buying a large amount of food, just make sure you are stocked with the basics like Jell-o, sugar-free Popsicles, broth, juice, Gatorade, mashed potatoes, soups, yogurt, grits and Cream of Wheat. You will eventually move into the protein rich foods and solids. Some surgeons start their patients off on protein supplements immediately.

Find out what your surgeon recommends for the first three weeks and buy those foods. You won't be eating very much, so don't purchase a lot.

Make Sure Your Home is Comfort Ready

If you have an open surgery, there will be some discomfort while those muscles and tissues are knitting back together. Consider purchasing a toilet seat lift and a shower chair. Your toilet at home will tend to sit lower than they are at the hospital. This won't be necessary if you have your surgery laproscopically. If you need to, rearrange your furniture and if you are too uncomfortable to climb the steps, set up a bed on the first level. If you have to climb the stairs to go to the bathroom, a portable toilet in case of emergencies might be helpful. Purchase extra pillows so that your bed will be comfortable. The hospital bed has controls, but your bed at home is lower and flat. Pillows will help make your bed more comfortable.

Take Enough Time Off Work

There is no need to rush back to a job when you have plenty of time to prepare for your absence. Carefully plan your absence so that the workplace doesn't need you for a while.

Double-Check Your Insurance Pre-Authorization

Check and double-check the wording of your pre-authorization. Make sure your surgery date is within the authorization window. Send or fax the pre-authorization to the surgeon, anesthesia group and hospital registration department. See if it is complete. Find out if you have to pay any fees before surgery. Ask if they take credit cards or personal checks. Once you pay, get a receipt! You may need to prove that you paid before surgery. Document, document, document! Document all of the instructions given to you by the surgeon, anesthesia group and the hospital.

Get Your Pre-Op Tests and Evaluations

Typical lab work, the EKG and X-rays are standard protocol for surgery. In most cases the tests have to be done within a 30-day window of your surgery date. Some surgeons require a Pap smear result, colonoscopy or other tests.

If you haven't had a psych evaluation, it may be required. Get it done and make sure that all your requirements are handled before surgery.

This is your journey. Stay on top of what you need done before your surgery date. Use the checklist at the end of this chapter or make up one of your own.

Pre-Op & Post-Op Medications

Get your prescriptions filled before your surgery. If you are self-paying, make sure you have at least enough medication filled to get you through the first two weeks post-op.

Durable Medical Power of Attorney & Will

Surgery is serious. Anytime you have surgery, please take the time to assign a Durable Medical Power of Attorney. This is a legal agreement that will allow someone to make decisions for you when you cannot. This person will have to abide by your written and stated wishes. Surgery will always carry some risk of death, even if it is minuscule, so checking over your will or making a will is truly important. I hope and pray that you will not need either. Surgery is safe, but you want to be responsible.

The Last Supper

Prior to surgery, many people eat like crazy. For the first time you may feel like you can eat anything and everything since your surgery is just around the corner. Since your new stomach can only hold a fraction of what it held before, this eating frenzy is a bon voyage party to your old stomach. The other reasons for eating like crazy is because you know you are going to be losing weight like crazy, so why not enjoy yourself while you can. Another reason is because you won't be able to tolerate anything beyond the soft diet for the first three weeks at least.

All I can say is enjoy this pre-surgery feasting time! Consider this time a glorious celebration of the new you soon to come, but be sure to stop your feasting a couple of days before surgery. Slow your intake to a lighter diet to allow your system to get cleaned out. Most surgeons will have you take a laxative as part of your pre-op medications. You will not be allowed to eat anything after midnight the night before your surgery.

Your recovery will be more comfortable if your system is cleaned out. So while your last suppers may be filled with every single sinful delight you can imagine, halt the celebration a couple of days before surgery.

Traveling For Surgery?

If you must travel for surgery, you have some special pre-surgery preparations.

Good Travel Planning

How are you going to get there and return home? Will it be by land, air or rail transit? Before making your reservations, double-check with the surgeon for the dates of your return. Arrive at least one full day in advance of your surgery or pre-op visit to the doctor. Check and see what restrictions are placed on your ticket in the event you need to stay longer than you expected. Consider the needs on your return trip. Long rides may tire you after surgery. So depending on how far you are traveling; the trip may need to be broken down into segments. If you are using air travel and you must change planes, tell your travel agent to make sure your layovers are at least an hour. You don't want to arrive at the airport and have to make a mad dash for the next flight, especially if you had the open surgery. Carry a bag with wheels to avoid heavy lifting and have someone help you with your luggage.

Book Your Hotel Room

The surgical group will probably have some suggestions about hotel accommodations and they may even have some discounts and special arrangements available to you. When you make your reservations, ask for a first floor room or a room near the elevator. You may want to avoid steps, especially if you had the open surgery.

Book Your Transportation

You will need some form of transportation whether it is from a cab service, shuttle or rental car. You may have some driving restrictions post-op. Have your transportation details ready before you arrive at your destination. Have your phone numbers and reservation numbers handy. Get a map and directions from the Internet or the surgical group. At a minimum you will need directions from the airport to the hotel, from the hotel to the surgeon's office and from the hotel to the hospital.

Pre-Surgery Preparation Check List

Here's a checklist to help you prepare for the big day!

☑	Item
	Take Pre-Op Pictures
	Start A Journal
	Take Pre-Op Measurements
	Align Support For Home & Family
	Clean The House Before Surgery
	Buy Your Food
	Make Sure Your Home is Comfort Ready
	Take Enough Time Off Work
	Double-Check Your Insurance Pre-Authorization
	Get Your Pre-Op Tests and Evaluations
	Fill Your Pre-Op & Post-Op Medication Prescriptions
	Prepare Your Durable Medical Power of Attorney & Will
	Book Your Travel Arrangements
	Book Your Hotel Room
	Book Your Transportation

Are You Fat or Food-Addicted?

Food is good. It looks good, smells good and tastes good. Food is associated with celebrations, holidays and good times. Everybody knows what it's like to eat until you're stuffed and uncomfortable. All you can do is unzip your pants, find a comfortable chair and plop down. This type of eating is not compulsive or impulsive overeating it's just overeating!

Addictive behaviors are compulsive and impulsive and food can be the drug of choice. Compulsive means to be compelled. When someone is compelled to eat, something is causing them to eat or something has occurred and it triggers the eating and in some cases overeating. The trigger could literally be anything and everything. Compulsive or obsessive behaviors can be anything from eating to gambling.

We know that eating more calories than are expended through

physical movement will generally lead to weight gain. Some compulsive, impulsive or obsessive overeaters may be fat.

The appropriate treatment for compulsive disorders is NOT bariatric surgery. Would you suggest that a gambler, alcoholic or spendaholic get bariatric surgery to cure their addiction to gambling, alcohol or spending? Absolutely not! Not all compulsive eaters are fat.

Compulsive eaters require treatment for how they respond to the triggers in their life, which sets off a chain of events that cause them or compel them to act out the problem behavior. The compulsive person needs help coping. The course of treatment may be psychological therapy, medication therapy or a combination.

Once this need to eat compulsively is under control, weight loss may occur as a result of less food intake. For the morbidly obese compulsive eater, weight loss may not occur even as a result of less food intake. Once the compulsive disorder is under control, bariatric surgery may be the treatment of choice to lose weight and keep it off.

The national guidelines for selecting a candidate for bariatric surgery include a psychological evaluation by a licensed psychologist or psychiatrist. It is important for the therapist to evaluate whether your eating is compulsive or "normal".

You may be thinking that you eat when you are nervous or when you are sad. In the Golden Girls sitcom, Dorothy, Sophia, Blanche and Rose would pull out the cheesecake anytime they had a problem. This is a normal behavior. We do use food to comfort us during a difficult time. The difference between using food as a normal coping mechanism and using it compulsively is probably how often and how much we use food to cope.

A compulsive eater that is not under control or left untreated will continue to compulsively eat after bariatric surgery. If you seriously think that you are a compulsive overeater, work with the psychologist or psychiatrist to resolve the compulsion first.

Chapter Ten

"Being fat is painful. And for fifty years I was fat. I have not been a normal sized person since I was seven years old. To those of you who are wondering if you should do this, ask yourself how many more years you want to live only dreaming of being normal, failing at yet another diet, beating yourself up emotionally because you believe you have failed at life because you cannot control your eating. I wish this had been an available option many years ago. Although I know wouldn't have been ready. I would have believed that the right diet was just around the corner. Don't do what I did. The years you are raising your children you need to be most active."

"Looks are just a small part of the damage morbid obesity does to you. It destroys your health and it destroys your self esteem. You are seeking, always, to work harder, faster, etc. just to feel that you are as good. You are always trying not to be classified as 'fat and lazy.' You don't want to be a stereotypical fat person."

"Near the end of this craziness, I no longer walked. I lumbered. I had a limp from all the damage that all the years and all the pounds did to my feet and legs and hips. I could wear only tennis shoes with orthotics. My hips hurt all the time. I had to look at chairs to see if they would hold me. When I had a chance to go somewhere, I had to worry about plopping half of me over into the next seat on an airplane, or face knowing that I did not fit through a turnstile."

"Today I am a normal sized person. No one looks at me and thinks I'm huge. I don't look at chairs first before I sit down. I'm not sexy, but that was not my motivation. I just wanted to stop hurting physically and emotionally. And I have. My wish for each of you would be that you can take the lesson I learned and apply it to your own life."

Florence Ballengee
http://www.geocities.com/tricia_810/mgb/indiv/flo.html
Laparascopic Billroth II, 5/31/2000

The Big Day!

This one day will change the rest of your life!

You will feel a mixed bag of emotions the morning of surgery. Fear, anxiety, excitement and relief are all common emotions. Some people find the emotions too overwhelming and back out. It doesn't happen often, but is has happened. If you've prepared yourself well, you won't have to worry. Many weight loss surgery patients adopt their surgery date as a second birthday. This shows just how significant "the big day" really is.

In this chapter, I am going to walk you through the big day, which actually starts the day before surgery. The day before surgery is just as important as the day of surgery.

One Day Before The Big Day

Try not to plan anything but your pre-surgical requirements on this day.

Packing For The Big Day

Have your bags packed by midnight the day before your surgery. At the end of the chapter, I'll provide a packing list for the big day.

Toiletry Items
Packing for the hospital is different from packing to go on vacation. All the basic toiletry items, except for shampoo, conditioner and deodorant, are all provided for you at the hospital. The hospital even supplies you with a toothbrush and denture cup. The brand of lotion, mouthwash, soap and toothpaste may be different from what you use at home, but for the short time you'll be at the hospital, you may as well use theirs. Although Vaseline is available, some people may want to take a lip balm.

Ladies, if you are on your cycle during surgery, pack some sanitary pads instead of tampons. Also pack big and roomy loose fitting underwear. Sometimes the hospital sanitary pads are the kind that must be worn with belts because they don't stock underwear.

Clothes
You won't need a change of clothes. The clothes you wear in the hospital are the same clothes you can wear home so make sure that you wear comfortable loose fitting clothes. Avoid zipper pants. Loose sweat suit type pants or a big billowy dress are good choices.

Gowns & Robes
The hospital provides gowns. Any hospital experienced in bariatric surgery will have gowns that are large enough for you. If they fit me, I'm sure they will fit you. Hospital gowns have a single tie at the neck and the sleeves have snaps. They are designed to make maneuvering around IV tubing and other tubes and drains easy. I don't recommend taking your own gowns because if they get soiled or stained from any drainage it just adds to your laundry when you get home. In addition, your own gown will be harder to manipulate with your IV and at dressing change time. You don't need to be a "fashion diva" in the hospital. The hospital gown is very practical for your stay. I also don't recommend taking your robe. Instead of using your own robe, use a second hospital gown as a robe. You can drape it around your shoulders so that the tie is at the front instead of the back.

Slippers
The hospital will provide "footies" with anti-skid rubber or tread on the bottom. If you don't want to walk around the hospital in them, you should take your own slippers. For those of you who have the open surgery, bending will be painful. You may want to take along the kind of slippers that you slip into instead of the kind that you have to pull on. The slip in type slipper exposes the heel.

Abdominal Binder
If you are having an open surgery, you want to check and see if the hospital will provide an abdominal binder. If not, then take your own. You can find an abdominal binder at the medical supply and equipment store. Make sure it fits before you leave the store. You may have to special order a size that fits correctly. Look in the phone book under "medical supplies". An abdominal binder will make you feel more secure as you start walking. If you are having laparoscopic surgery, you don't need an abdominal binder.

Money

Don't take any money with you to the hospital. My advice is to leave your purse and the usual purse and wallet items at home. Some hospitals charge a daily fee for the use of the television and others charge for the paper. If you take money for these things, you will not need over two or three dollars for each day. If you want to make long distance calls, you will need a calling card.

Jewelry

Don't take your jewelry. Remove all of your jewelry before going to the hospital and leave it at home.

Entertainment Items

The hospital stay can get pretty boring, so you may want to take along something to keep you busy. Books and magazines are a good choice. I don't recommend taking electronic items because they can be stolen. Unfortunately, theft happens everywhere.

Hospital Admission & Registration

I recommend that you pre-register at the hospital the day before your surgery. Waiting until the day of surgery can be a little nerve wracking. With all the emotions you experience on the day of surgery, you may be irritated with all of the admission processing, especially if there is a wait. Most hospitals allow pre-registering the day before your admission. During the admission process, the admitting clerk will make copies of your authorization letter, insurance cards and in some cases, your driver's license or other identification cards. You'll sign forms and the admitting clerk will go over some hospital information. More than likely, they'll give you a packet and some forms that you must present when you register for your surgery. If you want a private room, you need to request it at this time. There may be an extra fee. It may also affect whether you can have overnight guests in your room. You should ask about this during your registration. If you are a self-pay, you may be required to pay at the time of registration. The hospital usually requires a certified check. The registration process can take as little as fifteen minutes, but in some cases it can take up to an hour. If you don't pre-register the day before your surgery, make sure that you arrive at the hospital early to register. Some hospitals don't have a 24-hour registration desk. Therefore, you need to call the hospital to ask their registration hours. After hours registration is often done through the emergency room. Can you imagine the added stress of a morning mishap on the day of surgery? Pre-registration the day before surgery is a good idea.

What Time Is Your Surgery

Your surgeon will give you instructions about who and where to call to find out your surgery time. When you call, they will tell you your surgery time and when and where to report to the hospital. I recommend that you take a field trip to the pre-surgical area so that you won't be confused about where to report the day of your surgery. You can also map out where your family needs to park the day before surgery. All this preparation truly makes the day of surgery a breeze, especially if you are an out-of-towner. Don't you just love it when a plan comes together?

Your Diet The Day Before Surgery

Your food feast should have ended before this day. I recommend that you eat light. It will make your recovery more comfortable. The surgeon may have special diet instructions. If so, follow them. It is likely that one of your pre-op medications will include a laxative. The surgeon will want your system reasonably clean for surgery. It is a common surgical practice to prohibit you from eating or drinking anything after midnight the day before your surgery. You will be permitted to drink a sip of water if you have any pre-op medications before your surgery.

What About My Nails

The day before surgery, remove all of your nail polish. Your nails need to be bare; you should not wear clear nail polish. If you have acrylic or false nails, your surgeon will give instructions about them. The reason many surgeons will have you remove your false nails is because the anesthesiologist, doctors and nurses monitor the color of your nail beds to see if you are getting adequate oxygen. When you are getting inadequate oxygen, your nail beds turn a dark color. During surgery, an oxygen saturation monitor is placed on one of your fingers, usually the index finger. The monitor fits over your finger like a gentle clamp. If your nails are long, the monitor will not fit correctly. For this reason, you may be asked to cut at least the index fingernail short.

Pre-Op Medications

Each surgeon will have a pre-op medication schedule for you to follow. Follow it. If you are on additional medications the surgeon will also instruct you when to take those medications. When you are admitted to the hospital, the nursing staff will administer your medications by bringing them to your room. Pre-op medications for bariatric surgery will often include a laxative, an antibiotic and something for nausea. Your surgeon may also have you shower the morning of your surgery using a special skin cleanser. You should not take any anti-anxiety or relaxation medication until after you sign your surgical consent form the morning of surgery. The hospital must make sure that you are in your most conscious state when you give consent for surgery. If you are nervous at that time, they will give you something to relax you after you sign the consent form.

Practice Coughing & Deep Breathing Exercises

After surgery, you may get an incentive spirometer. This plastic apparatus is a tool that will help you deep breath. If you practice deep breathing exercises before your surgery, it will make it easier to deep breath after surgery. Deep breathing and coughing are very important for your circulation and lung function.

When To Go To Bed

You may be excited the night before your surgery. If you're like me, it was hard for me to fall asleep. You should probably not take a sleeping pill unless you have that cleared by your surgeon. Try as best as you can to get a good nights rest, at least eight hours of sleep the night before your surgery.

Finally! The Morning Of Surgery

If you are a morning eater, you may be hungry when you wake up. Out of habit, you may stumble to the refrigerator or coffee pot. If this is you, put a reminder note on the bathroom mirror and in the kitchen. "I AM NOT ALLOWED TO EAT OR DRINK ANYTHING."

If your pre-op medication schedule requires you to shower in a special anti-bacterial cleansing soap, your morning will start off with this activity. There may be instructions regarding shaving as well. After your shower, you will probably need to take your other pre-op medications. If you are well prepared, the only thing left to do is grab your bag and head to the hospital.

Pre-Surgery Check In

When you arrive at the hospital, have your family or support people hold onto your luggage. You'll need to check in at the pre-surgery desk. You need the paperwork given to you by the admission clerk when you registered. If you are the first surgery patient on the list, you won't have to wait in the pre-surgery waiting room. You'll be escorted to your pre-surgery room.

The Pre-Surgery Room

When it's your time for surgery, you'll be assigned a pre-surgery room. Your family will be able to join you in your pre-surgery room once the pre-surgery nurse gives the okay. The nurse will instruct you to remove all your clothes, place them in a plastic hospital bag, which is labeled with your name, and change into a surgical hospital gown and blue "lunch lady" cap. When you are in the cap and gown, the nurse will instruct you to make one last trip to the bathroom. After that, the nurse will take your height and weight measurements and check your vital signs. Someone from anesthesia along with the surgical nurse will verify and confirm any last minute information. You can also ask questions. A wristband with your name and your surgeon's name will be placed on your wrist. Make sure the information is correct. The last thing the surgical nurse will do is present you with the surgery consent form. The form outlines all of the surgical risks. You'll be asked to initial the pages and sign the form while the nurse witnesses your signature. If you sign the form without the nurse witnessing your signature, you may have to sign it again. The nurse then signs the consent form as a witness. After this processing, the surgical nurse will allow your family to join you in your pre-surgical room until it is time to go to surgery. When it's time for surgery, the nurse will have you lie down on the gurney and wheel you into the pre-operating room area. You'll say your farewells to your family. The next time you see them, you'll be post-op!

Pre-Operating Room Area

In the pre-op area your IV will be started and the anesthesia team will begin to give you medication to calm you. A good anesthesia nurse or doctor will deliver the medication slowly so that you won't get nauseated. You may want to ask them to deliver your medication slowly so that you won't get nauseated. When the surgery room is ready, you'll be wheeled into the operating room.

The Operating Room

You've probably seen an operating room (OR) before, even if it has been on television. The OR is cold. You'll be asked move from the gurney onto this narrow OR table. Its not very wide, but it is sturdy and it will support your weight. Once you are securely on the OR table, the OR nurse will place warming blankets over you. Underneath this blanket, your gown will be removed. The sides of the OR table have arm boards that extend out (sort of like a crucifix). You will relax your arms on the arm boards. The OR staff are usually very professional and they appear to have everything under control. They will secure you on this table with straps that gently secure your body and arms to prepare you for surgery. You may get a brief moment to say hello to your surgeon. Next, you'll be asked to breath into a plastic mask and that will be your last memory until you wake up in the recovery room. After your surgery, the surgeon will meet with your family in the waiting room and tell them the specifics of your surgery. If you don't want this meeting to occur, you have to notify your surgeon because meeting with the family after surgery is common protocol. Your family will be instructed to go to your hospital room and wait for you to arrive.

The Recovery Room

The recovery room nurses will let you wake up on your own or they may try to gently wake you. Most people wake up disoriented. It may take a second to get in your right mind. Most people wake up talking and confused about where they are. If you are in pain, the recovery room nurses will give you pain medication. They'll ask you how you feel, take your vital signs and keep you calm. After you are stable and comfortable, you'll be transferred to your room where your family will be waiting on you.

Your Hospital Room

You may be tired after surgery. I was. You are allowed to eat ice chips and clear liquids. Depending on your surgeon and surgery, you may have a urinary catheter. If you do, you won't have to get up and go to the bathroom. If you don't have a catheter, the IV fluids will have you running to the bathroom. Other than the trips to the bathroom, the first few hours after surgery are spent resting. It's unlikely that you'll want to entertain room guests this soon after surgery. Eventually though, you'll wake up, sit up and be more alert. As soon as you can, start walking. Walking and deep breathing exercises are the most important things to do after surgery and for the rest of your hospital stay. It can get pretty boring after a while. You will have a phone, television and whatever you brought along with you to keep you occupied and busy.

If you are in pain or nauseated, medication is just a call button away. Your hospital may have pain pumps that allow you to deliver your own pain medication. With each shift change, a nurse will visit you to assess how you are doing, check your vital signs, check your dressing and drainage tubes and clean and change your dressings. Depending on your surgery, you may not have any drainage tubes at all. Everyday your surgeon will visit you and check your status. Your diet for the full hospital stay will probably be clear liquids. This is pretty much the hospital routine for the rest of your hospital stay until you are discharged. Most laparoscopic patients are released within two days and most open patients have a five-day hospital stay.

Discharge Day

Discharges usually take place in the morning after breakfast, but before lunch. The nurse will go over your discharge instructions. If you still have a dressing upon the day of discharge, you should take home dressing supplies from the hospital so that you can change your dressings at home. Use your packing list to make sure you have all your belongings. When the nurse is finished completing your discharge process and paperwork, you will be free to pack your things and wait to be transported by wheelchair to the main entrance. Your family will meet you at the front door. It's now time to go home and start your post-op living.

☑ Big Day Checklist

The Packing List:

	Personal phone book
	Journal (to chronicle your WLS experience, thoughts and reflections)
	Deodorant (not perfume)
	Shampoo
	Conditioner
	Sanitary Pads & Big Roomy Underwear
	Slippers
	Abdominal Binder
	Money
	Calling Card
	Other Items

☑	**Pre-Registration List:**
	Insurance Letter and Pre-Authorization
	Certified Check (if needed)
	Driver's License
	Insurance Cards
	Durable Medical Power of Attorney Papers
	Private Room Request
	Questions about overnight guests
	Surgery Time and Reporting Detail
☑	**Pre-Surgery Preparation List:**
	Double-check your pre-op medications
	Reminder signs not to eat or drink
	Remove your nails and nail polish
	Eat light
	Practice deep breathing
	Get eight hours of sleep
☑	**The Morning of Surgery List:**
	Shower and shave
	Take your pre-op medications
	Wear big roomy loose fitting clothes
	Luggage
	Hospital admission paperwork from the registration
	Insurance cards
	Insurance letter and pre-authorization
	Driver's license

☑	**Last Minute Surgeon Questions:**
	Can I take anything to calm my anxiety?
	What pain medication will I be on after surgery?
	Will the hospital provide an abdominal binder?
	Can I take sleeping pills to help me sleep while in the
	Can I request a recliner chair in my hospital room?
☑	**Discharge List:**
	Your discharge instructions
	Dressing supplies
	Post–Op Medications
	Packing checklist to make sure you don't forget anything

Chapter Eleven

"I've been overweight all my life, and have been on doctor supervised diets since the age of six, and now at almost 16 years old. I'm nearing 300 pounds. I'm scared to think what my weight could be up to in the next few years if this pattern continues."

"I've been home schooled for the past few years because I was basically teased out of school. Until last year I couldn't even bare to get out in public. It seems like no matter how hard I try the weight just won't come off. My Mom has been one of my biggest supporters throughout the years. My Sweet Sixteen is coming up, and we were going to Disney World, but I ask my Mom to cancel the trip and save the money for my surgery. I wanted to go to Disney World, but I want to be healthy and fit more."

Mary Wester
Pre-op Laparascopic MGB

Post-Op Living

The First 18-24 Months Post-Op

Once you are home the first two or three weeks will be spent recuperating and adjusting. Even if you have the laparoscopic surgery and you're feeling great, your body is still in a recuperative state. Don't fool yourself.

While you are in the hospital the nursing staff will assess for possible complications, but when you return home you will need to assess yourself for possible complications. I suggest that you maintain a post-op journal. Even if you only want to jot down the date and a few words like "Recuperating well. Nothing unusual or out of the ordinary." It's better than nothing. Take your temperature everyday for the first ten days after returning home and keep a temperature record. If you experience complications, you want a record of when it started and how you felt. With any complication, you should contact your doctor, surgeon or hospital.

Post-Op Complications

Leaks

Leaks can occur at any of the new connection sites. The new connection sites are in the stomach and in the intestine. The chance of a leak is small. During surgery, the connections are tested using pressure to make sure there are no leaks, but the new connections are swollen at the time of surgery. As the internal swelling goes down, a leak can occur. The signs of a leak are a consistent and persistent abdominal pain. The pain can be dull or sharp. You can experience a burning or throbbing sensation and an increased temperature. Your abdomen may be warm to the touch. If you suspect you have a leak, go to the emergency room immediately. The emergency room will contact your surgeon. Leaks can be repaired, but they can also cause infection. Immediate treatment is important.

Pulmonary Embolism & Deep Vein Thrombosis

A pulmonary embolus is a blockage of an artery in the lungs. The blockage is caused by a blood clot. Blood clots invade the circulatory system when the blood gets too thick and clots are formed. Most pulmonary emboli are caused from clots originating in the lower legs. When the clots are in the lower leg, it is called a deep vein thrombosis. Clots sometimes resolve without treatment, but the general medical treatment is with blood thinners. A pulmonary embolism is extremely serious and can cause sudden death. Your risk for a pulmonary embolism or deep vein thrombosis increases with prolonged bed rest or inactivity after surgery. This is why deep breathing, walking and activity soon after surgery is so important.

The symptoms of pulmonary emboli aren't always alarming. It can be a cough that begins suddenly. You may produce bloody sputum with light blood streaks. You can have a sudden onset of shortness of breath at rest or with exertion. Lightheadedness, fainting and dizziness can also be a sign of a pulmonary embolism. The obvious signs are chest pain under the breastbone. The pain can be sharp, stabbing, burning and aching or a dull, heavy sensation that radiates.

Deep vein thrombosis can be caught by doing a simple test called the Homan's sign. While sitting up in bed, straighten both legs. Flex and point your toes towards your nose with your heels firmly planted on the bed. If you feel a sharp shooting pain in your leg, it is a positive Homan's sign. A positive Homan's sign is a strong indication that there's a deeply lodged clot. If you have these symptoms, you should go straight to the emergency room.

Incision Problems & Infection

Laparascopic incisions are so small that it is unlikely that they'll re-open, but it can happen. The open incision is more vulnerable to complications in the post-op phase. As you return home, clean your incision and observe the appearance. An infected incision will gape open, turn red, continue draining and will be warm and tender to touch. Some tenderness is expected, but the pain should be decreasing, not increasing. If an infection occurs, your temperature will increase. If you experience these problems or your temperature doesn't break, I suggest seeing the doctor as soon as possible.

The Post-Op Follow Up Visit

Sometime after your discharge, most bariatric surgeons will require a post-op office visit. During this visit, your surgeon will ask you questions, assess your condition, answer your questions, provide any additional information and remove your staples. If your incision is doing well, the reinforcement tape may not be needed. Sometimes this tape will cause skin irritation. Sometime during this visit, you will be pleasantly surprised. Your first official post-op weight will be taken and most people lose a significant amount of weight in just the first week. I lost 12 pounds by my post-op visit! Take your post-op journal and any list of questions with you. As your questions are answered, write down the answers.

Post-Op Medications

Some of your post-op medications will be short-term and others will be for a lifetime. The short-term post-op medications will typically include something for pain, something to reduce stomach acid and in some cases a preventative medication to avoid gall bladder problems. The long term or lifetime post-op medications are vitamins. Each surgeon will have a post-op medication schedule for you to follow and I suggest that you follow it.

Pain Medication
Depending on your type of surgery, you may not need any pain medication after discharge. Because your new smaller stomach is healing and part of your intestine has been bypassed, there are some pain medication restrictions. Most bariatric surgeons will advise you to avoid pain medications that contain ibuprofen, aspirin and acetaminophen. The reason is because these medications are hard on the stomach and can damage the stomach lining. The other reason is because there is less absorption of the medication in the intestine; the liver will have to work harder to detoxify the medication. Your surgeon will suggest a possible list of pain medications that are safe for you to take. For the rest of your life, you will need to keep a list of the medications that you should avoid. Give this list to your pharmacist and your PCP. There are many brand name medications that contain ibuprofen, aspirin and acetaminophen.

Acid Control
There are three types of acid control medications. They are antacids, like Tums, Rolaids, Mylanta and Maalox; acid controllers, like Pepcid, Tagamet and Zantac, and prescription proton pump inhibitors which stop the acid production, like Prevacid, Prilosec, AcipHex and Protonix. The stomach is a very acidic environment. But after surgery, this acidic environment can be difficult during the healing of the stomach. Therefore, acid control is necessary after surgery. You may also be prescribed Carafate, which protects the intestine from acid. Carafate is not an acid controller, but acts

as a coating for your stomach and intestine to protect the lining from acid and help aid in healing.

Bile Salts - Actigall
Actigall or ursodiol is used to prevent gallstone formation in people who are undergoing rapid weight loss. As mentioned earlier, some bariatric surgeons will remove the gall bladder to prevent gall stone formation. Others will prescribe this medication to preventatively stop gallstones from forming. If you don't have a gall bladder, you probably won't need to take ursodiol.

Vitamins
The body stores four vitamins. Vitamins A,D, E and K. The rest of the vitamins are not stored. Because you are losing weight rapidly, unable to eat as much due the smaller size of your stomach and the malabsorption of your bypassed intestine, you will need to take vitamins for life. There are a million vitamin choices on the market. Your surgeon will offer guidelines and instructions and I suggest you follow them.

Post-Op Diet

Your post-op diet will progress from clear liquids to solid foods over the course of three to six weeks. You don't have to be overly concerned with any special foods after weight loss surgery. Eating will soon return to a more "normal" pattern. Each surgeon has his or her own recommended diet with dietary restrictions. I suggest you follow it. I'm going to provide some basic nutrition information and guidelines to follow, not just in the immediate post-op phase, but also for the rest of your post-op life. Your new stomach will let you know if you are progressing too fast, eating too fast or eating too much.

The Importance of Protein
All food is made of carbohydrate, fat and protein. Carbohydrates are sugars. There are simple sugars and complex sugars. There are good fats and bad fats. And there are natural sources of protein and other sources of protein. Natural sources of protein come from meat, cheese and nuts.

Gastric bypass surgery causes weight loss and weight maintenance by reducing the amount of food consumed and reducing the amount of food absorbed. Food is absorbed in the intestine. The less intestine there is, the less food is absorbed in the intestine. A diet rich in protein is extremely important after gastric bypass surgery because less food is being absorbed. While carbohydrates and fats play an important role in the body, protein is necessary for every system in your body. Protein is necessary for cell growth and development. If you neglect to eat enough protein, you will feel and look weak. You must monitor your protein intake. Because your stomach is small, eating 50 or 60 grams of protein everyday can be difficult. Many post-op gastric bypass patients drink protein shake supplements. Whey and soy protein powders can be purchased at any nutrition store. You can probably find it in the grocery store. All shakes are not created equal. Learn to read the label and look for shakes that are protein based and not carbohydrate based. Ensure, Slim Fast and Carnation Instant Breakfast have high carbohydrate content. Read the label.

I recommend the book Sugar Busters. This book does a good job of describing the effects that sugar, fat and protein have on your body. The book suggests a diet high in protein, moderate in fat and low in carbohydrates.

Weight Loss Surgery Surprises - What To Expect

You will have to adjust to changes after surgery and if you are informed you will not be surprised. Some of the changes and adjustments are temporary and others are permanent. As you go through the list, know that not everyone will experience these "surprises." Surgery affects each person differently. There are many people who report that they haven't experienced anything from this list. I have found that knowledge and attitude have been the key to accepting or tolerating any of the changes whether they are temporary or long-term.

The Mental Adjustments

Head Hunger
Many obese people have no idea what real hunger feels like. Head hunger is more like a tempting thought or desire for food. It is a nagging suggestive head-trip. Head hunger is mental, not physical like real hunger pains. Head hunger can come about at anytime. Your brain does not know your stomach is a fraction of its original size. Your appetite may be suppressed after surgery, but it will return. When the appetite returns, the head hunger seems to come back with it. Head hunger will trick you into thinking that your new stomach can handle more than your stomach can hold. Head hunger will also have you eat something you know you can't handle. It can be somewhat depressing when your head hunger conflicts with your new stomach. Dealing with this is an adjustment.

Depression

In Chapter Nine, I dealt with some of the reasons you may experience depression. I strongly suggest that you find an accountability person to monitor your mood. This person can let you know if you seem to be slipping into some depressive moods. You will need support, but you may also need a counselor. Depression can be treated with psychotherapy, medication therapy or a combination. I do recommend though that before you begin taking antidepressants, check with your gynecologist to see if part of your depression is caused by a high level of free-flowing estrogen. The medication of choice might be hormone therapy and not antidepressants. The hormone imbalance will not last forever, it will resolve itself as the weight loss stabilizes.

"I'm Losing Too Slow"
Scale Stepping & Plateau Panic
Fear That Weight Loss Surgery Will Not Work For You

Weight loss can measured in many ways, but none more obvious than pounds. Weight loss can be measured in how many inches you lose and in how your clothes feel. For many people, myself included, weighing can become an obsession. I'm not going to offer advise on how often you should weigh yourself. Some people can weigh themselves daily and not panic about the reading, others cannot do this. I suggest that you honestly deal with how well you can cope when you weigh yourself. Especially when the pounds aren't coming off as fast as you want them to.

Weight loss plateaus are common and some people can't handle it. Nearly all weight loss surgery patients at one time or another have a fear that this attempt at weight loss through surgery will fail them just like the other diets and gimmicks. And who can blame you when every other thing you've tried has failed? Get to know yourself and bathe your mind in fact and not feelings. The fact is that you will more than likely lose 100 to 150 pounds in the first twelve months after surgery. The other fact is that you will have periods where your weight loss will plateau. The plateaus can even last a month or more. If you need to get rid of your scale at home, do so. In the moments when you start to feel anxious that weight loss is not happening fast enough, talk to a counselor or a supporter. You will not be the first person or last person to experience this anxiety and fear. It is one of the reasons why post-op support with other weight loss surgery patients is so vital. To help avoid "Plateau Panic" I've included a Plateau Panic worksheet in the Appendix on page 164.

I want to warn you not to compare your weight loss with others. Some people are able to lose weight more rapid than others. In my opinion, it appears that men seem to lose much faster than women. And the heavier you are, the faster the weight comes off, at first.

If you find that your weight loss is less than 100 pounds in the first 12 months, this would be considered a slower than average weight loss after gastric bypass surgery. This does not mean you will not continue to lose over the next 12 months. If you are in the less than 1% who experience poor weight loss after weight loss surgery, help is available through a surgical revision. You should not consider a revision before you are one year post-op. Do not be discouraged or disappointed if your surgeon will ask you to wait at least a year before considering a revision.

Fear About Stretching Your Stomach
There are times early in your post-op period that you may fear that you are "stretching your stomach." I suggest that you talk to your surgeon about how much stretching your new stomach will do over time. As time goes on this fear will subside.

When Food Was Your Friend (Or Enemy)
In Chapter Nine, I addressed "Are You Fat or Food Addicted." It is normal to use food as a short-term coping mechanism. We all have used food to help us though a moment of depression. If you have struggled with food addiction, you will need to continue with counseling because you will continue to eat after weight loss surgery. Binging will be more difficult due to the new size of your stomach. You can harm yourself mentally and physically if you slip back into old habits of compulsive eating.

Your Attitude About Exercise
It's a funny thing; weight loss surgery is likely to improve your mental outlook and attitude about exercise. Though exercise is not "required" after weight loss surgery, many of us start exercising because of the improved self-confidence and hope. I hated exercising before weight loss surgery because I associated exercise as just another failed attempt at weight loss. But now, I'm actually starting to like it and look forward to it.

The Estrogen Adjustments

Estrogen is stored in the fat cells. As you lose weight rapidly, estrogen is free-flowing. This free-flowing estrogen can create several significant problems: hair loss, contraceptive failure, fertility issues, depression, mood swings, nausea and period changes. Your gynecologist or PCP should monitor your estrogen levels. In some cases, you may need hormone therapy for a few months while the weight loss is the most rapid.

Hair Loss
Between months three and six, many weight loss surgery patients notice hair thinning and hair loss. I have never met anyone who went bald as a

result of weight loss surgery, but a few people who started out with very thin, fine hair have used wigs during this period. The cause of the hair loss is due to estrogen, but it can also be due to the rapid weight loss. The good news is that this is a temporary phase and most people report that once the hair shedding is over, the hair grows back faster, thicker and healthier. After monitoring literally thousands of emails about hair loss, the only suggestion I have to prevent making the situation worse is to give chemical treatments a rest between months three and six. Zinc tablets and hair vitamins don't seem to work for the people I've talk to. If you want to try them, they probably won't hurt, but they may not help.

Contraceptive Failure
This free-flowing estrogen will make hormone based contraceptive use ineffective. This would include the pill, injections and implants. The pill will likely fail during the time of your most rapid weight loss. Most bariatric surgeons will suggest that you delay getting pregnant for at least the first 18 months after surgery. Because of the estrogen release and the fact that hormone contraceptives won't work, you need to be very careful to find alternative methods of birth control.

Nausea
Nausea is common after weight loss surgery, but many people do not realize that the culprit may be estrogen. Nausea can often be corrected with temporary hormone therapy. If your nausea is not relieved with hormone therapy, you may need a medication for nausea.

Wacky Cycles
Many women report that their cycle is off for a while following weight loss surgery. Women report everything from a cessation of a period to abnormal periods. It is likely that this will reverse itself on its own when the estrogen levels stable out. Keep a record and discuss it with your gynecologist.

The Eating Adjustments

Some of the biggest adjustments you'll have to make will be in eating. Everything from what you eat to how much is all part of your new life. The longer you are post-op, the more you will know yourself and your new food limits, but the early post-op phase will be spent learning how, when and what to eat.

New Food Limits
One of the hardest things for me was adjusting to how to fix my plate. It seemed almost weird to fix a plate with just a tablespoon of this and that

on the plate, especially if it was a holiday meal. The plate looked empty, so I'd add more food on the plate, even though I knew I couldn't finish it. But then I started to feel like I was wasting food, and I hated to throw it out, so I'd wrap it up, but I don't like leftovers. Eventually, I accepted the smaller amount on my plate, but there were still food amount and limit issues that I had to adjust to, like restaurant dining. The restaurant portions are big even if you don't have surgery. Some people order from the kids menu, but not me. I find that kid menus are limited to chicken tenders and other finger foods. I wanted a real entrée. But I knew I'd only be able to eat a fraction of it. So doggie bags are a part of my post-op reality. And I still don't like leftovers. So I feel like I'm wasting money when I eat in a restaurant, but I'm slowly getting over it. You will also have test your new food limits and deal with the issues surrounding it.

Eating Slow & Chewing Well
Nearly all weight loss surgery patients have to learn a new eating pace. You will have to take smaller bites, chew well and eat slower. This new pace will be an adjustment if you were used to eating fast. As you eat slower, the temperature of your food will get cold. This was probably one of the hardest adjustments for me.

Food Intolerances
There are some foods that you ate before surgery that may not ever agree with your new stomach. For whatever reasons, when you take a bite or two of this "old favorite", your new stomach will simply not accept it. It may come up and out or it may just sit uncomfortably in your new stomach until the food passes. Either way, it can be difficult to say goodbye to an old favorite.

Changing Taste Buds
There's something about this surgery and your journey to wellness that can have a very positive effect. Before surgery, eating "right" may have been a challenge, but after surgery, there is a motivation that comes from the gained self-confidence as the pounds start to shed. Sometimes you just want to do something good for yourself, like making healthier food choices and exercising. Some people report that their taste buds actually begin to change and they enjoy a particular food that they didn't like before weight loss surgery.

Eating Without Drinking
Some people are unable to drink a beverage with their meal. They experience fullness much quicker if a beverage is part of the meal, even water. This can be a difficult adjustment for some. The larger your stomach pouch, the easier it is to tolerate a beverage with your meal.

The Physical Adjustments

There are several physical changes in addition to a shrinking body. There is the "dumping syndrome," halitosis, emesis and bowel changes.

Dumping
Dumping doesn't happen to everyone. I've never "dumped." Dumping is the result of eating foods high in simple carbohydrates, which in some will cause a hypoglycemic attack. Dumping can also happen if fluid is absorbed too quickly in the intestine. It seems to me that people without gastric bypass surgery can also "dump," but it's referred to as hypoglycemia. The symptoms of dumping include nausea, lightheadedness, weakness, fatigue, heart palpitations, clamminess, sweating, vomiting and diarrhea. If you are prone to dumping, it is important to figure out which foods trigger this event and once you find out, avoid them.

Emesis
Emesis means, "to vomit." Some things may not sit right in your new stomach. If you eat too fast, eat too much or eat something that doesn't agree with you, you may have some emesis problems. This should pass as you learn your new food limits and food tolerances. The emesis shouldn't be violent or gut wrenching. If something doesn't agree with your new stomach, your body will let you know right away.

Halitosis
A few post-op people have reported halitosis or bad breath. This could be attributable to a state of ketosis from a high protein, low carbohydrate diet.

Bowel Changes
Constipation is not likely to be a problem and neither should you experience diarrhea. Your stool will probably be softer, but formed. If you have issues with constipation or diarrhea, you will need appropriate treatment and investigation for why the problem is occurring. The frequency and urgency of your bowel patterns may also change. The color of your stool may be much lighter and depending on how much intestine was bypassed, you will absorb less fats and you may notice and orange residue in your stool. Lastly, many people report a significant change in the odor. Unfortunately, it is for the worse. I don't know if the smell is really worse, or if we just get used to smell of our own stool after so many years. Either way, it is likely that you'll notice an odor change. If you are self-conscious about the odor, carry matches. If you strike a match, the smell of the match overpowers the other scents. You are likely

to hear a variety of tips as you participate in support groups. I find that people are very creative.

Climate Sensitivity
Several post-op patients report being cold. This could be due to the hormonal changes. This tends to subside over time.

Losing Too Much Too Fast
I know it's hard to believe that losing too much or losing too fast could be a problem, but some people experience weakness if they lose too much too fast. If this is your case, your PCP should closely monitor you. You will need to be conscious about your vitamin supplements and protein intake.

Many people want to know how does the body know when to stop losing. I don't know how the body knows when to stop losing, but it does. Very few people experience so much weight loss that they have to have their surgery reversed or revised.

Dealing With The Restrictions

There are four primary restrictions after weight loss surgery.

Food Restrictions
Each surgeon will have a list of food restrictions. You may be given a list of foods to avoid. If you are obedient to the surgeon's recommended post-op diet, and one of your favorite foods is on the restricted list, you are likely to have a difficult time. Most of the food restrictions are not lifetime restrictions. Some surgeons instruct their patients to avoid beef for the first six months; others say nothing about avoiding red meat. There doesn't seem to be a consensus on food restrictions across the board. It seems to depend on your surgeon.

Medication Restrictions
I covered some of the post-op medication restrictions under Post-Op Medications earlier in this chapter. It is important for you to keep this list and provide it to your PCP and pharmacist along with a list of substitute medications to take in the place of the restricted ones.

Beverage Restrictions
There seems to be more consensus among the bariatric surgeons on beverage restrictions. Many will tell you to avoid coffee, tea and carbonated beverages, especially colas. The culprits seem to be caffeine and acid. These ingredients can irritate the lining of the stomach and intestine. These beverage restrictions can be difficult to follow if you are in the habit of drinking caffeinated and carbonated beverages.

Alcohol Restrictions

It is vital that you understand that alcohol is liver toxic. Because there is less intestine or "gut" to absorb food, the liver will have to work harder. Alcoholic beverages are more prone to cause liver dysfunction after gastric bypass surgery.

Dealing With The People

Two fairly large adjustments that you can expect are dealing with the comments and questions of people around you and knowing that you are being watched.

Comments & Questions

You will get comments and questions from anybody and everybody. Those who know you well will ask everything from how much you've lost to requests to see your incisions. If you don't want to show off your incision, kindly decline the request. Or if you are willing to "show and tell," consider showing photos of your incision if you are unable to show the real thing.

Even those who don't know that you had surgery can't help but comment as the weight starts to come off. Some people have tact, others don't. I suggest that you rehearse your answers because you will repeat them often. The people around you will have a natural curiosity. Some are rejoicing with you, others will be jealous of you. But this too will pass. As time goes on, you will mix in with the rest of the normal size people and the fact that you were once morbidly obese will no longer be the hot topic of conversation.

On Display

For the first year post-op, the people around you will watch you closely. They'll watch how you fix your plate, how much you eat, how slow you eat and what you eat. People are somewhat fascinated to see you change before their eyes and although you may not want to be "on display," you will be. Take pride in knowing that you have a life worth observing! Like the comments, the monitoring of your post-op behaviors will subside in time. Keep in mind that the same adjustments you are dealing with on the inside and outside are also shared by those around you. You have to get ready for a new you and so do they.

Chapter Twelve

"I have been overweight my whole life, but at 420 (BMI 72.1) I am at my highest weight ever. When I decided to have this surgery, my mother was less than enthusiastic, but agreed to support me in whatever way she could. I think telling her "Look Mom, I'm gaining weight while I talk to you" helped put where I am at in perspective."

"I get frustrated that I can't walk very far without getting out of breath or having my back hurt so bad that I have to stop and rest."

"Good luck to those of you thinking of having the surgery and God bless those of you that have."

Kymberleigh Warden
Open RNY, November 1999

Life After Surgery

24 Months & Beyond

At 24 months after weight loss surgery, most people will be at or near their goal weight. Sixty to eighty percent of the excess body weight should be gone for good without a fear of regaining it (as long as you exercise some good food choices). Some weight may return, but only a small amount. Don't panic, this is to be expected. Your weight will stable out as you settle into life as a normal size person.

The first two years after surgery were filled with victory after victory as the mental and physical burdens of being morbidly obese turn into memories. Some people report that they do a double take in a full-length mirror even years after weight loss surgery. The person staring back at them never takes the reflection for granted because they remember a day when looking in that full-length mirror was torture. And others report that they are tempted to tell morbidly obese people on the street about the help available through weight loss surgery.

At the two-year mark, you have an entirely new wardrobe for your new body. As you settle into your normal size body, you will meet people who never knew the "morbidly obese you." And even when you share the story and show photos, they will stare in disbelief.

Even though your body is a normal size, you cannot become lax or too comfortable and forget that your body has been anatomically altered. The consequence of weight loss surgery is an agreement for long-term follow-up and restrictions.

The Lifetime Agreements

Vitamins & Minerals
For the rest of your life, you need to take your vitamins and minerals. You will always be at a higher

risk of developing nutritional deficiencies due to the malabsorption of food. As long as you remain compliant with your supplements, you should be fine.

Giving Blood
Some bariatric surgeons suggest that you abstain from being a blood donor due to the iron therapy required and the malabsorption in the intestine.

Endoscopes
Add an endoscopy test to your annual physical. Like a mammogram or a Pap smear, the endoscopy test is a preventative measure. It will reveal any potential complications with the digestive system.

Annual Blood Work
Every year you should have a complete blood count and a full chemistry panel. Any nutritional deficiencies will be revealed in these tests.

Medication Restrictions
Your restrictions are a lifetime commitment. Always notify your pharmacy and PCP of your medication restrictions. Some people have elected to wear a medic-alert bracelet. This is your choice. If you are not compliant with the medication restrictions, you are at risk for liver dysfunction and gastric problems.

Lifelong Support
Expect a gradual transformation from needing support to lending support. The longer you spend time in your normal size body, the more you will spend time enjoying it. And that means less time for participating in the support groups. Just remember, the "newbies" need you.

Continue Exercising
It's not "required," but exercise is good for you.

Pregnancy
After the first two years, if you choose to have children, remember to notify your obstetrician that you had gastric bypass surgery. You will probably need to take a greater amount of nutritional supplements and have your blood tests done more frequently as a precaution.

The Transformation Continues - Cosmetic Surgery
Improving On A Good Thing (The Plastic Doctor)

The term plastic surgery comes from the Greek word "plastikos" which means, "to mold." Many weight loss surgery patients embark on a second phase of their body transformation with plastic surgery. Several of the bariatric surgeons suggest that you wait 18 months to two years before considering plastic surgery. You can learn more about plastic surgery on-line at http://www.plasticsurgery.org and http://www.dryoho.com. Dr. Yoho has an entire book available on-line.

Removal Of Excess Skin

Sagging skin isn't attractive and you may elect to have it nipped and tucked in various places. Don't buy into the rumor that the burn center will pay for plastic surgery in exchange for your excess skin.

Liposuction

Those nagging fat deposits that won't go away regardless of your weight loss can be removed with a liposuction. Body contouring and reshaping can be done from head to toe.

Arm Lift (Brachioplasty)

This is the name of the surgery that gets rid of those "bat wings." You know, the skin that hangs down on your upper arms.

Tummy Tuck (Abdominoplasty)

Also known as panniculectomy, abdominal sculpting can be achieved using different techniques. I have found the most extraordinary photos on-line at http://plasticsurgery4u.com. If you are queasy about medical photos, don't look.

Breast Lift (Mastopexy)

Need I say more?

Thigh Lift

Need I say more?

Butt Lift

Need I say more?

In Conclusion

Writing this book has been a pleasure. I want you to enjoy every single day of the rest of your life! God bless you as you embark on your journey to wellness and freedom from obesity.

Appendix

What WLS has done for me...

"Hope is the whole-hearted belief that something GREAT is going to happen. It is the joyful anticipation of a fulfilled end in your favor. Hope is a close cousin to faith. I think that the best thing that the weight loss surgery has done for me is given me hope to overcome the trappings of obesity."

Michelle Boasten

Appendix

NATIONAL INSTITUTES OF HEALTH
National Heart, Lung, and Blood Institute
NHLBI Communications Office (301) 496-4236
Press Release: Wednesday, June 17, 1998

First Federal Obesity Clinical Guidelines Released

The first Federal guidelines on the identification, evaluation, and treatment of overweight and obesity in adults were released today by the National Heart, Lung, and Blood Institute (NHLBI), in cooperation with the National Institute of Diabetes and Digestive and Kidney Diseases (NIDDK).

These clinical practice guidelines are designed to help physicians in their care of overweight and obesity, a growing public health problem that affects 97 million American adults – 55 percent of the population.

These individuals are at increased risk of illness from hypertension, lipid disorders, type 2 diabetes, coronary heart disease, stroke, gallbladder disease, osteoarthritis, sleep apnea and respiratory problems, and certain cancers. The total costs attributable to obesity-related disease approaches $100 billion annually.

"Overweight and obesity pose a major public health challenge. The development of these guidelines was a pioneering achievement since they were the first ever developed by the Institute using an evidence-based model and methodology," said NHLBI Director Dr. Claude Lenfant. "This report will be an invaluable clinical tool for any health care professional who works with overweight or obese patients," he added.

The guidelines are based on the most extensive review of the scientific evidence on overweight and obesity conducted to date. The review involved a systematic analysis of the published scientific literature to address 35 key clinical questions on how different treatment strategies affect weight loss and how weight control affects the major risk factors for heart disease and stroke as well as other chronic diseases and conditions.

The guidelines present a new approach for the assessment of overweight and obesity and establish principles of safe and effective weight loss. According to the guidelines, assessment of overweight involves evaluation of three key measures– body mass index (BMI), waist circumference, and a patient's risk factors for diseases and conditions associated with obesity.

The guidelines' definition of overweight is based on research which relates body mass index to risk of death and illness. The 24-member expert panel that developed the guidelines identified overweight as a BMI of 25 to 29.9 and obesity as a BMI of 30 and above, which is consistent with the definitions used in many other countries, and supports the Dietary Guidelines for Americans issued in 1995. BMI describes body weight relative to height and is strongly correlated with total body fat content in adults. According to the guidelines, a BMI of 30 is about 30 pounds overweight and is equivalent to 221 pounds in a 6' person and to 186 pounds in someone who is 5'6". The BMI numbers apply to both men and women. Some very muscular people may have a high BMI without health risks.

The panel recommends that BMI be determined in all adults. People of normal weight should have their BMI reassessed in 2 years.

"The evidence is solid that the risk for various cardiovascular and other diseases rises significantly when someone's BMI is over 25 and that risk of death increases as the body mass index reaches and surpasses 30," said Dr. F. Xavier Pi Sunyer, chairman of the expert panel and director of the Obesity Research Center, St. Luke's/Roosevelt Hospital Center in New York City.

"The guidelines tell the truth about the risks associated with unhealthy weight. We hope that physicians and the public will take the message seriously and use the guidelines to begin to deal effectively with a difficult problem," asserted Dr. Pi-Sunyer.

According to a new analysis of the National Health and Nutrition Examination Survey (NHANES III), as BMI levels rise, average blood pressure and total cholesterol levels increase and average HDL or good cholesterol levels decrease. Men in the highest obesity category have more than twice the risk of hypertension, high blood cholesterol, or both compared to men of normal weight. Women in the highest obesity category have four times the risk of either or both of these risk factors.

The guidelines recommend weight loss to lower high blood pressure, to lower high total cholesterol and to raise low levels of HDL or good cholesterol, and to lower elevated blood glucose in overweight persons with two or more risk factors and in obese persons. Overweight patients without risk factors should prevent further weight gain, advise the guidelines.

In addition to measuring BMI, health care professionals should evaluate a patient's risk factors, such as elevations in blood pressure or blood cholesterol, or family history of obesity-related disease. At a given level of overweight or obesity, patients with additional risk factors are considered to be at higher risk for health problems, requiring more intensive therapy and modification of any risk factors.

Physicians are also advised to determine waist circumference, which is strongly associated with abdominal fat. Excess abdominal fat is an independent predictor of disease risk. A waist circumference of over 40 inches in men and over 35 inches in women signifies increased risk in those who have a BMI of 25 to 34.9.

According to the guidelines, the most successful strategies for weight loss include calorie reduction, increased physical activity, and behavior therapy designed to improve eating and physical activity habits. Other recommendations include:

Patients should engage in moderate physical activity, progressing to 30 minutes or more on most or preferably all days of the week.

Reducing dietary fat alone–without reducing calories–will not produce weight loss. Cutting back on dietary fat can help reduce calories and is heart-healthy.

The initial goal of treatment should be to reduce body weight by about 10 percent from baseline, an amount that reduces obesity-related risk factors. With success, and if warranted, further weight loss can be attempted.

A reasonable time line for a 10 percent reduction in body weight is six months of treatment, with a weight loss of 1 to 2 pounds per week.

Weight-maintenance should be a priority after the first 6 months of weight-loss therapy.

Physicians should have their patients try lifestyle therapy for at least 6 months before embarking on physician-prescribed drug therapy. Weight loss drugs approved by the FDA for long-term use may be tried as part of a comprehensive weight loss program that includes dietary therapy and physical activity in carefully selected patients (BMI >30 without additional risk factors, BMI >27 with two or more risk factors) who have been unable to lose weight or maintain weight loss with conventional non-drug therapies. Drug therapy may also be used during the weight maintenance phase of treatment. However, drug safety and effectiveness beyond one year of total treatment have not been established.

Weight loss surgery is an option for carefully selected patients with clinically severe obesity – BMI of > 40 or BMI of >35 with coexisting conditions when less invasive methods have failed and the patient is at high risk for obesity-associated illness. Lifelong medical surveillance after surgery is a necessity.

Overweight and obese patients who do not wish to lose weight, or are otherwise not candidates for weight loss treatment, should be counseled on strategies to avoid further weight gain.

Age alone should not preclude weight loss treatment in older adults. A careful evaluation of potential risks and benefits in the individual patient should guide management.

According to NHANES III, the trend in the prevalence of overweight and obesity is upward. The guidelines note that from 1960 to 1994, the prevalence of obesity in adults (BMI >30) increased from nearly 13 percent to 22.5 percent of the U.S. population, with most of the increase occurring in the 1990s.

"There are several possible reasons for the increase," asserted Karen Donato, coordinator of the Obesity Education Initiative. "When people read labels, they're more likely to notice what's low fat and healthy but may not be looking at calories. Also, more people are eating out and portion sizes have increased. Another issue is decreased physical activity. So people are consuming more calories and are less active. It doesn't take much to tip the energy balance," she said.

The upward trend in adult obesity has also been observed in children, notes the report. Since treatment issues surrounding overweight children and adolescents are quite different from the treatment of adults, the panel called for a separate guideline for youth as soon as possible. However, a healthy eating plan and increased physical activity is an important goal for all family members.

With that in mind, the guidelines contain practical information on healthy eating. Based on this material, the NHLBI has developed consumer tips on shopping, eating, and dining out.

The guidelines have been reviewed by 115 health experts at major medical and professional societies. They have been endorsed by the coordinating committees of the National Cholesterol Education Program and the National High Blood Pressure Education Program, the North American Association for the Study of Obesity, the NIDDK Task force on the Prevention and Treatment of Obesity, and the American Heart Association. These groups represent 54 professional societies, government agencies, and consumer organizations. Clinical Guidelines on the Identification, Evaluation, and Treatment of Overweight and Obesity in Adults will be distributed to primary care physicians in the U.S. as well as to other interested health care practitioners. It is available on the NHLBI Website. Single free copies of the consumer tips referred to above are available by writing to the NHLBI Information Center, P.O. Box 30105, Bethesda, MD 20824-0105.

National Institute of Health Obesity Report
282-Page Full Report on the Clinical Guidelines on the Identification, Evaluation, and Treatment of Overweight and Obesity in Adults from the NIH
* http://www.nhlbi.nih.gov/guidelines/obesity/ob_home.htm

BMI Calculators on the Internet
Website Addresses
* http://www.nhlbisupport.com/bmi
* http://www.insweb.com/health/tools/bmi.htm
* http://www.clos.net/bodymassindex.htm
* http://www.obesityhelp.com/morbidobesity/bmi-start.phtml
* http://www.nhlbi.nih.gov/guidelines/obesity/bmi_tbl.htm

Metropolitan Height & Weight Table For Men

Height	Small Frame	Medium Frame	Large Frame
5' 2"	128-134	131-141	138-150
5' 3"	130-136	133-143	140-153
5' 4"	132-138	135-145	142-156
5' 5"	134-140	137-148	144-160
5' 6"	136-142	139-151	146-164
5' 7"	138-145	142-154	149-168
5' 8"	140-148	145-157	152-172
5' 9"	142-151	148-160	155-176
5' 10"	144-154	151-163	158-180
5' 11"	146-157	154-166	161-184
6' 0"	149-160	157-170	164-188
6' 1"	152-164	160-174	168-192
6' 2"	155-168	164-178	172-197
6' 3"	158-172	167-182	176-202
6' 4"	162-176	171-187	181-207

Metropolitan Height & Weight Table For Women

Height	Small Frame	Medium Frame	Large Frame
4' 10"	102-111	109-122	118-131
4' 11"	103-113	111-123	120-134
5' 0"	104-115	113-126	122-137
5' 1"	106-118	115-129	125-140
5' 2"	108-121	118-132	128-143
5' 3"	111-124	121-135	131-147
5' 4"	114-127	124-138	134-151
5' 5"	117-130	127-141	137-155
5' 6"	120-133	130-144	140-159
5' 7"	123-136	133-147	143-163
5' 8"	126-139	136-150	146-167
5' 9"	129-142	139-153	149-170
5' 10"	132-145	142-156	152-173
5' 11"	135-148	145-159	155-176
6' 0"	138-151	148-162	158-179

The Plateau Panic Chart

Along the second to left hand column, enter the date one week from your surgery date. For example, if your surgery was 1/1, the week 1 date will be 1/8, the week 2 date would be 1/15. In the third column, "Total Pounds Lost", enter the cumulative amount of pounds you've lost. So if you lose 10 pounds by the end of week 1, write in 10, and if you lose 5 pounds by the end of the second week, write in 15.

The numbers to the right reflect the cumulative amount of pounds you can expect to lose by the end on the week. Some people will lose 100 pounds over the year and others will lose 180 pounds or more. This chart is different from the expected weight loss chart your surgeon will provide to you. This chart amortizes your weight loss over the full year. It is designed to help you keep some perspective during your plateaus. There's nothing more frustrating than those plateaus.

Week	Date	Total Pounds Lost	100 Pound Loss	120 Pound Loss	140 Pound Loss	160 Pound Loss	180 Pound Loss
1			2	2	3	3	3
2			4	5	5	6	7
3			6	7	8	9	10
4			7	9	11	12	14
5			10	12	14	15	17
6			12	14	16	18	21
7			13	16	19	21	25
8			15	18	22	25	28
9			17	21	24	28	31
10			19	23	27	30	35
11			21	25	30	34	38
12			23	28	32	37	42
13			25	30	35	40	45
14			27	32	38	43	49
15			29	35	41	46	52
16			31	37	43	49	55
17			33	39	46	52	59

Week	Date	Total Pounds Lost	100 Pound Loss	120 Pound Loss	140 Pound Loss	160 Pound Loss	180 Pound Loss
18			35	41	49	55	62
19			37	44	51	58	66
20			38	46	54	61	69
21			40	48	56	64	73
22			42	51	59	68	76
23			44	53	62	71	80
24			46	55	65	74	83
25			48	58	68	77	87
26			50	60	70	80	90
27			52	62	73	83	93
28			54	64	76	86	97
29			56	67	78	89	100
30			58	69	81	92	104
31			60	71	84	95	107
32			62	74	86	98	111
33			63	76	89	101	114
34			65	78	92	104	118
35			67	80	95	107	121
36			69	83	97	111	125
37			71	85	100	114	128
38			73	87	103	117	132
39			75	90	105	120	135
40			77	92	108	123	138
41			79	94	111	126	142
42			81	97	113	129	145
43			83	99	116	132	149
44			85	101	118	135	152
45			87	104	122	138	156
46			89	106	124	141	159
47			90	108	127	144	163

Week	Date	Total Pounds Lost	100 Pound Loss	120 Pound Loss	140 Pound Loss	160 Pound Loss	180 Pound Loss
48			92	110	130	147	166
49			94	113	132	150	170
50			96	115	135	154	173
51			98	117	138	157	177
52			100	120	140	160	180

Sample Diet History

Use this chart as a guideline to help you assemble your diet history. In the first column, enter the name of the diet you tried. In the second column, enter the date or year. In the next column, enter the name of your PCP during this time. Then enter the pounds lost, if any pounds were lost and in the last column enter your comments. The comments can include anything you remember about being on this diet. Were you on this diet alone, with friends, was it supervised by your physician, how long were you on this diet and did you gain the weight back.

Name of Diet	Date, Year	Physician	Pounds Lost	Comments

Sample Letter

Letter from the PCP and/or Surgeon to the Insurance Company

Dear Sir or Madam:

This is a formal request for pre-approval and pre-authorization for gastric bypass surgery, CPT-4 Code [enter code here] for [name of patient]. Morbid obesity is a lethal disease that kills hundreds of thousands of Americans every year. You will find that [patient name] meets all of the nationally recognized guidelines for the surgical treatment and intervention for morbid obesity.

Physician	Name & Title; Address; Phone; Fax
Member	Patient Name: Social Security Number: Address: City, State, Zip: Phone Number: Insurance Carrier: Group/Policy/Member Number:
Attention	Please Note: This is NOT a Cosmetic Procedure. The requested surgery is medically necessary. The patient meets Milliman and Robertson Guidelines for the Surgical Treatment of Morbid Obesity.
Height	[Enter height]
Weight	[Enter weight]; Based upon the Metropolitan Life Insurance table of desired weight, this patient should be [enter desired weight]. This patient is morbidly obese carrying an extra [enter pounds] pounds of excess weight.
BMI	[Enter BMI]
Waist	[Enter Waist Circumference]
Obesity-Associated Illnesses	[List all obesity-associated illnesses]
Enclosures	Diet History; Surgical Candidacy Checklist; Medical Record

Obesity Guidelines from Milliman and Robertson

- At least 100 pounds over the ideal weight as defined by the Metropolitan Life tables or the patient must have a body mass index exceeding 40. Or if the body mass index is 35, there must be a clinically serious condition like obesity hypoventilation, sleep apnea, diabetes, hypertension,

cardiomyopathy or musculoskeletal dysfunction.
- The patient must show that they have failed to lose weight significantly or has regained weight despite compliance with a multidisciplinary non-surgical programs including a low or very low calorie diet, supervised exercise, behavior modification and support.
- The patient should not have any correctable cause for obesity like an endocrine disorder.
- The patient must be full-grown and have reached full growth.
- The patient should be treated in a surgical program with experience in obesity surgery, including, not only surgeons experienced with gastric bypass, but also a multidisciplinary approach including all of the following: preoperative medical consultation and approval, preoperative psychiatric consultation and approval, nutritional counseling, exercise counseling, psychological counseling and support group discussions.

Patient Assessment

Chief Complaint	Morbid Obesity (ICD9 Code 278.01); [Include other obesity-associated diagnosis with ICD-9 codes]
History of Present Illness	[Enter patient information]
Medications	[Enter patient information]
Allergies	[Enter patient information]
Alcohol; Smoking	[Enter patient information]
Family History	[Enter patient information]
Musculoskeletal	[Enter patient information]
Respiratory	[Enter patient information]
Cardiovascular	[Enter patient information]
Digestive Disease	[Enter patient information]
Genitourinary	[Enter patient information]
Gynecologic	[Enter patient information]
Endocrine	[Enter patient information]
CNS	[Enter patient information]
Overall Assessment	[Enter patient information]
Impression and Plan	
Referring MD	Dr. Name; Practice Name & Specialty; Address; City, State, Zip; Phone Number; Fax Number

Sample Letter

Letter from Psychiatrist or Psychologist to Insurance Company or Referring Physician

Dear Sir or Madam:

According to the national guidelines for the surgical intervention for the treatment of morbid obesity, I find that [patient name] is a good candidate for gastric bypass surgery.

- This patient is aware of the adjustment to the side effects of the surgery.

- This patient is aware of the potential for serious complications, the associated dietary restrictions, and the occasional failures.

- This patient is committed to lifelong medical follow-up.

I recommend [patient name] for the surgical treatment for morbid obesity.

Sample Letter

Personal Letter to the Insurance Company
(can be used on first request or with an appeal)

Dear Medical Directors/Review Committee:

This letter comes in response to my request for a surgical solution to my lifelong struggle with obesity. Please allow me to tell you about my history and myself as well as educate you about Weight Loss Surgery.

I am a [enter age] year-old morbidly obese [enter gender]. It is my dream to live as any normal size person and get off of this up and down dieting roller coaster that has plagued my life since age [enter age]. I am unable to [enter physical burdens associated with your obesity]. This has created so much shame in my life that only other morbidly obese people can truly understand the humiliation.

While I am not mentally ill, I do have mental burdens associated with being morbidly obese. [Include mental burdens].

All of these problems can be helped by losing weight. I have tried many, many diets. (I have included my diet history with this letter.) While I have lost weight before on different diets, the weight just comes back, sometimes more. I am [enter weight] pounds and without surgical intervention, I think that I will die soon and the medical professionals all agree. My BMI is [enter BMI], that makes gastric bypass surgery a medical necessity.

I am very well educated in the area of Gastric Bypass Surgery. I have been researching this procedure, and its incredible success rate for [enter time]. I have been attending support group meetings to become well acquainted with others who also suffered at the hands of morbid severe obesity. I also belong to an on-line support group. I have learned a tremendous amount from all these people. I know what this surgery is and what positive implications it will have in my life. That is why I want and need to have this surgery. After reviewing my family medical history, you will probably agree with me that to not have this surgery will surely lead to more severe medical problems in the NEAR future.

My PCP, surgeon, and my counselor all agree that this procedure is the right option for me. I also agree with them. I want this surgery. It will save my life, and give me back what life I have left. I will not give up on getting this procedure approved. I will keep coming back. However, if this surgery request is denied, I will not be coming back alone. I have already spoken with an attorney, who will be representing me if the need be. So, I beg you, please approve this surgery. I will not go away. This surgery is as critical as a coronary bypass graft or neurosurgery. It is the ONLY documented long-term solution to chronic morbidly severe obesity. I am greater than 100 pounds over any recommended table. The Metropolitan Height and Weight Tables prove this.

I don't know your medical background, but some physicians are unaware about the great amount of research that has been conducted. The American Medical Association studies that have been published in JAMA well document that surgical intervention is the treatment of choice for the morbidly obese. The misconception about this surgery by those unaware of the disease of morbid obesity is that it is a cosmetic procedure. Let me assure you that this is completely false. I have taken the liberty of going to the American Society for Bariatric Surgery (ASBS) website and the National Institute of Health's website to gather information for you. You will quickly see that there is NOTHING cosmetic about this procedure.

Clinically severe (Morbid) obesity correlates with a Body Mass Index (BMI) of 40 kg/m2 (or higher) or with being 100 pounds overweight. Being overweight is associated with real physical problems, which are now well recognized. The most obvious is an increased mortality rate directly related to weight increase.

Obesity is dangerous to health because of the associated increased prevalence of cardiovascular risk factors such as hypertension, diabetes mellitus, hypertriglyceridemia, hyperinsulinemia and low levels of high-density lipoprotein (HDL) cholesterol. Cardiovascular risk factors are reduced significantly by sustained weight reduction. Data from the Framingham study support the estimate that a ten percent reduction in body weight corresponds to a twenty percent reduction in the risk of developing coronary heart disease.

The risk for diabetes has been reported to be about twofold in the mildly obese, fivefold in moderately obese and tenfold in severely obese persons. The risk of developing diabetes also increases with age, if a family history is present and if the obesity is central.

Surgical treatment is medically necessary because it is the only proven method of achieving long-term weight control for the severely obese. Surgical treatment is not a cosmetic procedure. Surgical treatment of severe obesity does not involve the removal of adipose tissue (fat) by suction or excision. Bariatric surgery involves reducing the size of the stomach, with a degree of associated malabsorption from bypassed intestine. Eating behavior improves dramatically.

Weight reduction surgery has been reported to improve several co-morbid conditions such as glucose intolerance and diabetes mellitus, sleep apnea and obesity-associated hypoventilation, hypertension, and serum lipid abnormalities. A recent study showed that Type II diabetics treated medically had a mortality rate three times that of a comparable group who underwent gastric bypass surgery. Also preliminary data indicate improved heart function with decreased ventricular wall thickness and decreased chamber size with sustained weight loss. Other benefits observed in some patients after surgical treatment include improved mobility and stamina. Many patients note a better mood, self-esteem, interpersonal effectiveness, and an enhanced quality of life. They have lessened self-consciousness. They are able to explore social and vocational activities formerly inaccessible to them. Self body image disparagement decreases.

For many reasons, I am a good candidate for this surgery and I ask you to approve me for gastric bypass surgery.

Department of Insurance Contact Information

State	Phone No.
Alabama	(334) 269-3550
Alaska	(907) 465-2515 (907) 269-7900
Arizona	(602) 912-8444 (520) 628-6371 (800) 325-2548
Arkansas	(800) 852-5494 (501) 371-2640
California	(800) 927-4357 (213) 897-8921 (800) 967-9331 (916) 322-3555 (415) 904-6072
Colorado	(303) 894-7499 (303) 894-7490 (303) 894-7495

State	Phone No.
Connecticut	(800) 203-3447 (860) 297-3800
Delaware	(302) 739-4251
Florida	(850) 413-3100 (800) 342-2762
Georgia	(404) 656-2070 (800) 656-2298
Hawaii	(808) 586-2790
Indiana	(317) 232-5251
Idaho	(208) 334-4250
Illinois	(217) 782-4515 (312) 814-2427
Iowa	(515) 281-5705
Kansas	(800) 432-2484

State	Phone No.	State	Phone No.
Kentucky	(800) 595-6053 (502) 564-3630	North Dakota	(800) 342-4718
		Ohio	(800) 686-1526
Louisiana	(225) 342-5900 (800) 259-5300 (800) 259-5301	Oklahoma	(405) 521-2828 (800) 522-0071
Maine	(207) 624-8475 (800) 300-5000	Oregon	(800) 542-3104 (503) 373-1692
Maryland	(410) 468-2017	Pennsylvania	(877) 881-6388
Massachusetts	(617) 521-7794	Rhode Island	(401) 222-2246
Michigan	(877) 999-6442 (517) 373-0220	South Carolina	(803) 737-6160
		South Dakota	(803) 737-6160
Minnesota	(651) 297-7161	Tennessee	(615) 741-1900
Mississippi	(800) 562 2957 (601) 359 2453	Texas	(800) 252-3439
		Utah	(801) 538-9674
Missouri	(573) 751-4126	Vermont	(800) 917-7787 (802) 863-2316
Montana	(800) 332-6148		
Nebraska	(402) 471-2201	Virginia	(800) 552-7945 (804) 371-9741
Nevada	(775) 687-3370 (702) 486-3587 (888) 333-1597	Washington	(360) 664-2879
		West Virginia	(304) 558-7000 (888) 558-7002
New Hampshire	(603) 271-2261	Wisconsin	(608) 266-3585 (800) 236-8517
New Jersey	(800) 838-0935		
New Mexico	(505) 827-4601	Wyoming	(307) 777-7344
New York	(212) 480-6400	Washington D.C.	(202) 724-5626
North Carolina	(800) 546-5664 (919) 733-2032		

On-Line Support Groups

http://groups.yahoo.com/group/MiniGastricBypass
http://groups.yahoo.com/group/OSSG
http://www.obesityhelp.com/morbidobesity/chatroom.phtml
http://nav.webring.yahoo.com/hub?ring=wlssring&list
http://www.myminigastricbypass.com/SupportGroups.htm
http://clubs.yahoo.com/clubs/gastricbypasspeople
http://clubs.yahoo.com/clubs/afterweightlosssurgery

May I Pray With You?

prayer (prår) noun.

A reverent petition made to God, a god, or another object of worship.

The act of making a reverent petition to God, a god, or another object of worship.

An act of communion with God, a god, or another object of worship, such as in devotion, confession, praise, or thanksgiving.

A specially worded form used to address God, a god, or another object of worship.

A religious observance.

A fervent request.

The thing requested.

The slightest chance or hope.

My Prayer For The Person Struggling With Morbid Obesity

I thank you Lord for the genetic composition that made me who I am. You created me and you knew full well what was wrong with me. I thank you for each person that teased me, rejected me, laughed at me and talked about me. While it hurt, these experiences made me strong and taught me how to forgive and love despite the persecution. I thank you because I understand pain and it has made me empathetic to the plight of anyone else in pain. I cannot turn away as if I don't understand emotional anguish. This experience has taught me compassion and humility. It has also taught me discernment. I am truly grateful for that. Being overweight was a small price to pay to learn what I have learned. The experience has been invaluable. I thank you Lord that you were my comfort when no one else could comfort me. This made me depend on you and lean on you more and more. My faith has been increased because of this.

Thank you that I didn't lose my mind when I knew that there was more going on inside my body when everyone else thought it was "just food". Lord you confirmed this for me before I learned about the genetic research. I am grateful to you for imparting the surgeons and the researchers and the medical community with the wisdom, insight and knowledge to unravel some of your great mysteries about our bodies that are fearfully and wonderfully made.

For each person making the decision to have weight loss surgery, I pray for a successful surgery and recovery. Lord steady the hands of the surgeons, give them peace and a confident assurance as they try to help someone overcome the physical affliction of morbid obesity. Steady the nerves of those undergoing the surgery that they may have peace and rest by knowing that you are our Sovereign God and NOTHING happens to us without you allowing it to happen. We know that everything works together for the good to those who love you and are called according to your purpose.

Lastly Lord, if the reader is unsaved, I pray that they will come to know you and grow in their salvation.

Amen

More WLS Books are on line at www.alongtheweigh.com

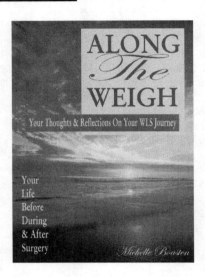

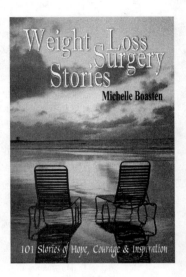

Along The Weigh
ISBN 1-931033-02-1

Along The Weigh: Your Thoughts & Reflections on Your WLS Journey - Your Life Before, During & After Surgery is the companion journal to Weight Loss Surgery: Understanding & Overcoming Morbid Obesity. This 154-page book and photo journal is designed for you to chronicle your weight loss surgery story before, during and after surgery in words and photos.

The journal will help guide your thoughts. It will assist you in documenting your journey so that it is organized and thorough. You will never regret keeping your story well documented. It is part of the healing journey and it will make an incredible keepsake as you share your story with others and encourage them in their own WLS Journey.

Weight Loss Surgery Stories
ISBN 1-931033-03-X

Weight Loss Surgery Stories: 101 Stories of Hope, Courage & Inspiration is like "Chicken Soup for the WLS Soul." You are not alone in your WLS Journey. This journey has been traveled by many people. Reading their stories will surely give you encouragement.

I would not have had the courage to share my own story had it not been for many others who shared theirs. Nothing could replace the support and encouragement I found in knowing that I was not alone. Someone could related to what I was going through.

This book is for anyone at any point in their WLS Journey.